Blood Donors and the Supply of Blood and Blood Products

Forum on Blood Safety and Blood Availability
Division of Health Sciences Policy
INSTITUTE OF MEDICINE

Frederick J. Manning and Linette Sparacino, *Editors*

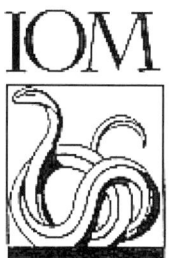

NATIONAL ACADEMY PRESS
Washington, D.C. 1996

National Academy Press 2101 Constitution Avenue, NW Washington, DC 20418

NOTICE: The project that is the subject of this report was approved by the Governing Board of the National Research Council, whose members are drawn from the councils of the National Academy of Sciences, the National Academy of Engineering, and the Institute of Medicine. The members of the forum responsible for this report were chosen for their special competencies and with regard for appropriate balance.

This report has been reviewed by a group other than the authors according to the procedures approved by a Report Review Committee consisting of members of the National Academy of Sciences, the National Academy of Engineering, and the Institute of Medicine.

The Institute of Medicine was chartered in 1970 by the National Academy of Sciences to enlist distinguished members of the appropriate professions in the examination of policy matters pertaining to the health of the public. In this, the Institute acts under both the Academy's 1863 congressional charter responsibility to be an adviser to the federal government and its own initiative in identifying issues of medical care, research, and education. Dr. Kenneth I. Shine is president of the Institute of Medicine.

Support for this project was provided by the Food and Drug Administration (Contract No. 223-93-1025), Abbott Laboratories, Baxter Health Care Corporation, Ortho Diagnostic Systems, the American Association of Blood Banks, the American Red Cross, the American Blood Resources Association, and the Council of Community Blood Centers. This support does not constitute an endorsement of the views expressed in the report.

Library of Congress Catalog Card No. 96-69896
International Standard Book Number 0-309-05577-6

Additional copies of this report are available from: National Academy Press, Lock Box 285, 2101 Constitution Avenue, N.W., Washington, DC 20055. Call (800) 624-6242 or (202) 334-3313 (in the Washington metropolitan area), or visit the NAP on-line bookstore at **http://www.nap.edu/nap/bookstore**.

Call (202) 334-2352 for more information on the other activities of the Institute of Medicine, or visit the IOM home page at **http://www.nas.edu/iom**.

Copyright 1996 by the National Academy of Sciences. All rights reserved.

Printed in the United States of America

The serpent has been a symbol of long life, healing, and knowledge among almost all cultures and religions since the beginning of recorded history. The image adopted as a logotype by the Institute of Medicine is based on a relief carving from ancient Greece, now held by the Staatlichemuseen in Berlin.

Cover design by Francesca Moghari.

FORUM ON BLOOD SAFETY AND BLOOD AVAILABILITY

HENRIK H. BENDIXEN, *Chair*, Professor Emeritus, Department of Anesthesiology, Columbia University, New York, New York.
THOMAS F. ZUCK, *Vice Chair*, Professor of Transfusion Medicine, University of Cincinnati, and Director, Hoxworth Blood Center, Cincinnati, Ohio
JOHN W. ADAMSON, President, New York Blood Center, New York, New York
ARTHUR L. CAPLAN, Director, Center for Bioethics, University of Pennsylvania, Philadelphia, Pennsylvania
WILLIAM COENEN,* Administrator, Community Blood Center of Greater Kansas City, Kansas City, Missouri
PINYA COHEN, Vice President of Quality Assurance and Regulatory Affairs, NABI, Boca Raton, Florida
EDWARD A. DAUER, Dean Emeritus, College of Law, University of Denver, Denver, Colorado
M. ELAINE EYSTER, Distinguished Professor of Medicine, Division of Hematology, The Milton Hershey Medical Center, Hershey, Pennsylvania
JOSEPH C. FRATANTONI, Director, Division of Hematology, Office of Blood Research and Review, Food and Drug Administration, Rockville, Maryland
HARVEY G. KLEIN, Chief, Department of Transfusion Medicine, Warren Grant Magnuson Clinical Center, National Institutes of Health, Bethesda, Maryland
EVE M. LACKRITZ, Medical Epidemiologist, HIV Seroepidemiology Branch, Division of HIV/AIDS, National Center for Infectious Diseases, Centers for Disease Control and Prevention, Atlanta, Georgia
PAUL R. McCURDY, Director, Blood Resources Program, National Heart, Lung, and Blood Institute, Bethesda, Maryland
PAUL S. RUSSELL, John Homans Professor of Surgery, Massachusetts General Hospital, Boston, Massachusetts
CAPT BRUCE D. RUTHERFORD, MSC, USN, Director, Armed Services Blood Program, Falls Church, Virginia
WILLIAM C. SHERWOOD, Director, Transfusion Services, American Red Cross Blood Services, Philadelphia, Pennsylvania
LINDA STEHLING, Director of Medical Affairs, Blood Systems, Inc., Scottsdale, Arizona

---

* Served from January 1995 until December 1995.

EUGENE TIMM,** Member, Board of Directors, American Blood Resources Association, Rochester Hill, Michigan

ROBERT M. WINSLOW, Adjunct Professor of Medicine, University of California-San Diego, and Hematology-Oncology Section, Veterans Affairs Medical Center, San Diego, California

Project Staff

VALERIE P. SETLOW, Director, Health Sciences Policy Division
FREDERICK J. MANNING, Project Director
KIMBERLY KASBERG MARAVIGLIA, Research Associate
MARY JANE BALL, Senior Project Assistant
NANCY DIENER, Financial Associate (until March 1996)
JAMAINE TINKER, Financial Associate (after March 1996)

** Served from January 1994 until December 1994.

PRESENTERS

DAVID V. BONK, Director of Membership, Marketing, and Public Relations, Blood Bank of Delaware, Newark, Delaware

ARTHUR BRACEY, Transfusion Services, St. Luke's Episcopal Hospital, Houston, Texas

JEFFREY L. CARSON, Professor and Chief, Division of General Internal Medicine, Robert Wood Johnson School of Medicine, University of Medicine and Dentistry of New Jersey, New Brunswick, New Jersey

LLOYD COHEN, George Mason University School of Law, Arlington, Virginia

ALVIN DRAKE, Ford Professor of Engineering, Massachusetts Institute of Technology, Cambridge, Massachusetts

ROBERT FIELDS, Manager, Meat Merchandising and Procurement, Kroger Company, Cincinnati, Ohio

JOSEPH C. FRATANTONI, Director, Division of Hematology, Office of Blood Research and Review, Food and Drug Administration, Rockville, Maryland

RONALD GILCHER, Oklahoma Blood Institute, Oklahoma City, Oklahoma

COLONEL JOHN HESS, MC, USA, Blood Research Detachment, Walter Reed Army Institute of Research, Washington, D.C.

JEANY MARK, Director, Strategy, Policy and Analysis, Biomedical Services, American Red Cross, Arlington, Virginia

JEFFREY McCULLOUGH, Director, Clinical Labs, University of Minnesota Hospital, Minneapolis, Minnesota

TOBY SIMON, President, Blood Systems Foundation, Scottsdale, Arizona

DOUGLAS SURGENOR, Senior Investigator, Center for Blood Research, Boston, Massachusetts

C. ROBERT VALERI, Naval Blood Research Laboratory, Boston, Massachusetts

COLONEL MICHAEL J. WARD, BSC, USAF, Industrial College of the Armed Forces, National Defense University, Washington, D.C.

ROBERT G. WESTPHAL, Blood Services, Northeast Region, American Red Cross, Dedham, Massachusetts

FOREWORD

This is the second in a series of three monographs by the Forum on Blood Safety and Blood Availability. Each monograph provides a review and summary of selected topical presentations at four separate workshops sponsored by the Forum from January 1994 through September 1995. The previous volume dealt with the Forum's discussions of governmental regulation of blood banking and was entitled *Blood Banking and Regulation: Procedures, Problems and Alternatives*. A future volume on safety and risk collects the Forum's discussions of transfusion-related disease transmission and related topics. The talks summarized in this document were originally given at a workshop on blood availability held in Washington, D.C., on June 8 and 9, 1995. The views expressed in this document, unless otherwise noted, are those of the individual presenters and do not reflect the views of the individual's employing agency or the Institute of Medicine. To promote full participation by Forum members, presenters, and invited guests, the Forum does not draw conclusions or make recommendations.

The Forum on Blood Safety and Blood Availability was convened by the Institute of Medicine to provide a nonadversarial environment where leaders from the private blood community, the Food and Drug Administration (FDA), academia, and other interested parties could exchange information about blood safety and blood availability, identify high-priority issues in these areas, and promote problem-solving activities such as workshops. Although the inclusion of FDA officials among its members precluded the Forum from giving advice or making recommendations, during its two years of existence, the Forum identified opportunities and problems that are ongoing or expected to arise within the next five years, and has explored approaches to exploiting opportunities or solving problems.

During the final meeting, in September 1995, members of the Forum reviewed its work and addressed the question of how the dialogue that it had fostered might best be continued or improved. One of the questions the group considered was what the criteria should be for any such future venture. Not everyone agreed with everything mentioned, and no votes were taken; consistent with its charter, the Forum reached no specific conclusions or recommendations. The group did, however, request that the collected list of criteria be recorded as a possible starting point for any subsequent initiative. The suggestions on that list included the following "Criteria for a Process of Dialogue:"

1. A consensus oriented procedure capable of reaching closure on the issues being discussed.
2. Participation of diverse constituencies, such as designated representatives the public.
3. Continuity of people and process, so that issues may be addressed as they arise without the need to fashion a structure and process ad hoc.
4. Conditions supporting openness and candor.
5. Opportunities for discussion in a variety of venues, both public and —where permitted by law—private.
6. Prestigious and neutral, a forum that lends dignity and credibility to the discussions.
7. Expert facilitation, though not necessarily subject-matter expertise, by those who run or manage the process.
8. Less time devoted to education about the issues, allowing more direct engagement with decision-making.
9. Available and ready to be utilized whenever an appropriate issue is identified.
10. Fashioned to be persuasive to Congress and others.

PREFACE

For a decade after the emergence of transfusion-associated AIDS, the overriding concerns with the American blood supply have centered on risk. Blood centers and hospital blood banks have been viewed less as guardians of the blood supply than as guarantors of its safety. Few members of the general public, or of the medical profession for that matter, worry much about the availability of blood. Surgeons and patients alike expect compatible blood to be available when they want it and in an amount sufficient to meet the immediate need.

For the most part, these expectations have been met. Adequacy of supply and availability of blood for all Americans are, after all, two of the four goals of our National Blood Policy of 1973. Supply and access hold equal status with the principles of blood safety and system efficiency. Why then has the country experienced serious blood shortages during the past two years, and is this situation likely to worsen during the next decade?

Supplying blood to patients throughout the United States turns out to be a more complicated issue than most people realize. Blood is collected by a patchwork system of large and small blood centers and hospitals and distributed by a variety of local and national mechanisms. Collections have been further subdivided into those from anonymous community donors, (allogeneic blood), donations from patients for their own use (autologous blood,) and allogeneic blood collected from friends and relatives for a specific patient (directed donations). There is also a parallel system of paid plasma donation which is used for manufacturing a variety of blood derivatives. Surprisingly few hard data are available concerning the supply of blood components from year to year, let alone from month to month and day to day. Even less is known about how blood is used. We have preconceived notions about when to expect blood shortages, but there are regional differences as well as differences in the blood type in short supply. None of these is as well understood as many believe. Are we barely able to collect all the blood that we need, or do collectors intentionally limit the amount of blood they collect—and occasionally fail to estimate accurately? Are we really running short of blood donors because of changing donor demographics and attitudes and increased deferral of donors during the screening process? Some argue that there are plenty of donors and opportunity to increase the number of donations, but that the system, despite years of study, still fails to attract and retain these donors. Others believe that we have learned little about distributing blood in an effective and efficient manner and that better management of our current collections could easily eliminate shortages. Still others look to science to provide longer blood storage intervals, less expensive cryopreservation, or blood substitutes as answers to the fluctuating supply problem.

Furthermore, the system is changing. We are experiencing a rising competition for donors and blood that has not been seen for a quarter of a century. Regional suppliers have become national suppliers. Hospitals and HMOs exert substantial financial pressures as they seek the best price for their blood services. Would the American public be better served by a monolithic system of collection and distribution like that which many European countries have established? Could we improve supply and cost without sacrificing safety by replacing a system based on altruistic blood donation with one based on paid donation? Is blood a "national resource," or is that just a euphemism for a not-so-special perishable commodity, much like vegetables or seafood? How would this perception affect the public's willingness to donate blood?

With these questions and many more in mind, the Forum on Blood Safety and Blood Availability convened several panels to explore several of the issues involved in blood supply. Among the participants were well-known students of the American system of supply and distribution, custodians of the blood inventory at the hospital, regional and national levels, and individuals with expertise in recruitment and inventory management from outside the discipline of blood transfusion. The presentations and discussions proved illuminating.

This monograph represents the deliberations of a one-day workshop on blood availability. It seemed obvious a priori that not all of the questions, let alone the answers, could emerge from one such gathering. In fact, our meeting focused almost exclusively on whole blood and red blood cells, although platelets and white blood cells are major aspects of transfusion medicine as well. If a few additional insights into these issues of national importance have resulted from this workshop, however, it will have served its purpose.

HARVEY G. KLEIN
WORKSHOP MODERATOR

CONTENTS

I	**Current State of the Blood Supply**	1
	Longitudinal Studies of Blood Availability, *Douglas M. Surgenor*,	3
	Blood Supply Fluctuations, *Jeffrey McCullough*,	9
	When Should Physicians Transfuse? *Jeffrey L. Carson*	19
	International Perspectives on Blood Availability, *Robert G. Westphal*,	25
II	**Enhancing Collections**	31
	The Delaware Plan, *David Bonk*,	33
	Markets and the Blood Supply, *Lloyd Cohen*,	41
	Blood Donor Attitudes and Behavior, *Alvin Drake*,	45
III	**Enhancing Distribution**	51
	American Red Cross Blood Distribution System, *Jeany Mark*,	53
	Blood Resource Sharing Programs, *Toby Simon*,	59
	Exporting Blood from a Regional Blood Center, *Ronald Gilcher*,	65
	Supply and Demand in Transfusion Services, *Arthur Bracey*,	71
	Logistic Problems and Perishables: The Kroger Company and Supermarket Seafood, *Robert Fields*,	77
IV	**Expanding the Alternatives**	81
	Frozen Red Cell Technology, *C. Robert Valeri*,	83
	Logistical Concerns in Prepositioning Frozen Blood, *Michael J. Ward*,	91
	Extended Liquid Storage of Red Blood Cells, *John Hess*,	99
	Overview of Blood Substitutes, *Joseph Fratantoni*,	103

V	**Closing Remarks**	107
	Henrik H. Bendixen,	109
	Harvey Klein,	111
	Appendixes	115
A	Acronyms,	117
B	Workshop Participants,	119

I
CURRENT STATE OF THE BLOOD SUPPLY

Longitudinal Studies of Blood Availability

Douglas M. Surgenor

I will present some findings today from a survey of blood collections and transfusions in the United States during the 1992 calendar year.[1]

Blood is collected by two types of institutions in the United States: regional blood centers and hospitals. In 1992, estimated domestic blood collections included 12,035,000 units of allogeneic blood, i.e., blood donated by others; 1,117,000 units of autologous blood, i.e., blood donated by patients for their own expected use; and 436,000 units of directed blood, i.e., blood donated by others for use by designated patients (Table 1). Most of the domestic blood (approximately 90 percent) was collected by 176 regional and community blood centers. The remainder was collected by hospitals. Testing of blood for disease and other markers resulted in the exclusion of 4.5 percent of collected units.

When 1992 collections were compared against 1989 collections, some interesting trends were noted. Total estimated allogeneic collections decreased by 7.0 percent. On the other hand, autologous donations increased by more than 70 percent, while directed donations increased by almost 25 percent. The strong upward trend in autologous and directed donations reflects patient concerns about the safety of the blood supply. The high rates of nonutilization of these units are attributable to overdonation beyond expected need, lack of clear criteria for their transfusion, and hesitancy to "cross over" unused units for use by others. Unfortunately, there is a large economic cost to the nonutilization of these units; in many instances, the cost must be borne by the hospital in which the units were not transfused. We observed substantial differences between the rates of autologous and directed donations in different U.S. census regions. In New England, autologous units represented 3.2 percent of total collections, and in the Pacific region, autologous units represented 9.9 percent of total collections. The high rate in the Pacific region has been

---

[1] A more detailed report of this survey is available in Wallace, EL, WH Churchill, DM Surgenor, J An, G Cho, S McGurk and L Murphy (1995). Collection and transfusion of blood and blood components in the United States, 1992. *Transfusion, 35:* 802–812.

attributed, in part, to legislation in California that requires counseling of patients about their transfusion options. Similar differences were observed in the rates of directed donation, from 0.8 percent in New England to 6.1 percent in the East South Central region.

TABLE 1 Units of Red Blood Cells (RBC) and Platelets Collected and Transfused in the United States in 1989 and 1992.

Blood Component	1989	1992	% Change
Collected			
Allogeneic RBC	12,939,000	12,035,000	-7.0
Autologous RBC	655,000	1,117,000	70.5
Directed RBC	350,000	436,000	24.6
Platelets	2,190,000	3,828,000	74.8
Transfused			
Allogeneic RBC	11,532,000	10,491,000	-9.0
Autologous RBC	356,000	566,000	59.0
Directed RBC	97,000	136,000	40.2
Platelets (apheresis)	2,112,000	3,642,000	72.4
Platelets (concentrate)	5,146,000	4,688,000	-8.9

Transfusions of blood and its components were given almost exclusively to hospitalized patients. Transfusions of allogeneic blood fell by 9 percent between 1989 and 1992. This was the first time in over 20 years of surveillance of the national blood supply that such substantial declines in these indices of transfusion activities have been recorded. The U.S. red cell transfusion rate, measured in units transfused per thousand population, also fell substantially. The proportion of collected units of red cells that were transfused varied depending on donation category. Approximately 92 percent of collected allogeneic units remaining after testing were transfused. However, only 51 percent of autologous units were transfused to the patient who gave them. The remaining autologous units were not used. As for directed units, only 31 percent were transfused.

The findings from this survey indicate that over 1.5 million units of allogeneic red cells from the national blood resource were outdated, lost, or unaccounted for during 1992 (Table 1). Given a red cell dating period of about 35 days, this implies that 100,000 units of red cells became outdated every 35 days during the year. Most of those units were on hospital blood bank shelves when they became outdated. Assuming that every allogeneic unit had an equal chance of being transfused to a patient, this corresponds to an average of 20 units of various blood types becoming outdating every 35 days in each of 5,000 hospitals.

The high rate of non-use of autologous and directed units (49 percent) stems from the fact that such units were only rarely used for unrelated patient transfusions.

Our observations on the collection and transfusion of platelets are of particular interest. Collections of apheresis platelets increased by more than 72 percent between 1989 and 1992. Apheresis is a procedure in which, using a special machine, blood is collected, platelets are separated, and the remaining parts of the blood are returned to the donor. Apheresis platelets so obtained are called single donor platelets to distinguish them from pooled platelet concentrates that are separated from donated whole blood from many donors. The data in Table 1 also reveal substantial changes in the sources of the platelets that were transfused. Between 1989 and 1992, transfusions of single donor platelets increased by more than 72 percent. In the same period, transfusions of platelet concentrates decreased by almost 9 percent in the same interval. The result was a substantial increase in the proportion of platelets being transfused as single donor (apheresis) platelets. This trend benefits patients who need platelets by reducing donor exposure, risks of infection, and immunization and transfusion reactions.

QUESTIONS AND COMMENTS

Alvin Drake: Doug, of the people who give autologously in preparation for their surgery, any idea of how many of those people end up getting blood from the common supply anyway because the autologous donation wasn't enough?

Douglas Surgenor: It is an interesting problem. In a cohort of over 500 total hip replacement patients who had predeposited autologous units, we observed that the proportion of patients who completely avoided transfusion with allogeneic units increased as the number of units predeposited increased from one up to four units. About 80 percent of the patients who donated two units avoided any allogeneic transfusion. When three units had been donated, about 95 percent avoided allogeneic transfusion. However, there was an offsetting cost: the percentage of donated autologous units that were not needed rose from about 20 percent when two units were predeposited to 50 percent when three units were predeposited.

Toby Simon: If I followed your discussion correctly, the outdate or discard rate on allogeneic, undirected, and non-autologous blood is in the neighborhood of a million units. Not included in that is a discard rate from directed and autologous donations, so your actual discard rate is close to 1.9

million units a year?

Douglas Surgenor: Yes. That is about right.

Arthur Bracey: I am very interested in that 1.9 million units. Are there data reported by the hospital transfusion services to the AABB on outdates so that you can compare the calculated number with the observed number?

Douglas Surgenor: A large proportion of the data that we used to estimate the national activities that I have touched on came from reports submitted to AABB by its member hospitals.

William Sherwood: There seems to be a focus on that 1.9 million outdates and the study, I am assuming, did not number these by blood type. It would be my observation that these outdates are mostly Type A and Type B and if anyone is looking at these as a source to solve a nationwide problem of occasional shortages, that really won't be useful. Our shortages are usually Type O, and distributing more of those Type A's and Type B's around the country isn't going to help.

Douglas Surgenor: That is a good point. We found that if you take autologous and directed units out of the picture and just look at the difference between what allogeneic blood was collected and what was transfused in 1989 and 1992, the same net amount of blood was not used. It comes out at about a million units that were not used in each year. That suggests there is kind of an irreducible minimum.

Eve Lackritz: What I found interesting is you are seeing an increase in these directed and autologous donations, which is being driven, perhaps, by concerns about the safety of the general supply. But in actuality, you say the blood supply is getting progressively safer over the years.

Douglas Surgenor: That is a fact, but we don't know the factors that may be driving autologous and directed donations.

Ernest Simon: I think the point you made is that there were a million units that are unaccounted for. It is not clear that they are outdated. The reason I mention that is that I think in the Booz-Allen report of 1971, there was about 25 percent that was unaccounted for. And I am not sure that we should equate "unaccounted for" with "outdated."

Douglas Surgenor: No, the point being that you have got to realize that the blood resource is spread over these several thousand hospitals in the United States. In addition to actual outdating, there is loss due to breakage, handling, and that sort of thing.

Celso Bianco: Dr. Surgenor, you implied that it was somewhat unfair for the patient's hospital to be charged for all of these units that are ultimately not used. Who should pay for them?

Douglas Surgenor: I don't know. All I know is that there is an inequity here that hasn't been addressed.

Harvey Klein: As you pointed out, these data were collected in 1992. There were enormous trend changes between 1989 and 1992. We don't know what is happening between 1992 and 1995. Do you know of any effort to collect such data? Are you going to be collecting them, or do you know of any efforts to get more rapid turnaround so that we can make decisions more reasonably, based on available data.

Douglas Surgenor: Yes. We have initiated a new survey of collections and transfusions. With the cooperation of AABB, we hope that the results can be made available by 1996.

Blood Supply Fluctuations

Jeffrey McCullough

This presentation will focus on fluctuations in the blood supply. First of all, why should we care about the fluctuation in the blood supply? An inadequate blood supply may pose a danger to patients if the proper amount and type of blood is not available when needed. It may lead to longer hospital stays if elective procedures must be postponed in order to wait for an adequate blood supply. This leads to increased costs, as well as potential risks for patients. On the other hand, an excess supply leads to wastage and increased costs, and it also calls into question whether we have served blood donors properly by obtaining blood that is not needed or was not used for patient therapy.

Is there a problem with the fluctuation in the blood supply, and if so, how big is the problem? Acquiring these kinds of data is fairly difficult, so the data are not as adequate as would be ideal in order to address this issue. Hospitals usually track blood utilization in fairly large blocks of time, quarterly or monthly. Although the data are available, it is not customary for hospitals to look at fluctuations in blood usage on a weekly or a daily basis. Thus, by looking at utilization data in a longer time frame, some of these fluctuations don't become apparent. What we are really concerned about is more short term fluctuations in the blood supply that will lead to temporary imbalances.

Today I am focusing on short-term fluctuations, where it is necessary to tailor the blood availability to specific patient needs. Over the longer term, there will be shifts in blood utilization based on changes in medical therapy and changes in the indications for transfusion, leading to variations in the blood supply. The blood supply that is necessary in a hospital is based on physician requests for blood to be made available for use rather than actual blood use. The size of the inventory is thus not necessarily based on how much patients use. If requests for blood are far in excess of actual usage, the hospital's inventory is inflated and the likelihood of blood wastage then increases. This is something that we dealt with over the last 15 years with the development of more structured approaches to the amount of blood that is crossmatched.

There is some need for an extra safety margin in the blood inventory. One of the issues is the size of this safety supply or safety margin. Is it possible to have this safety margin without some outdating or wastage? It may be that this kind of a safety stop is necessary in order to operate the system.

I want to look at the extent of this fluctuation and spend a few minutes talking about the reasons for these kinds of fluctuations and how well the system is organized to cope with these fluctuations. The average weekly blood usage from our hospital, the University of Minnesota Hospital, from May 1, 1994 through May 1995 was 264 units of red cells (Figure 1). The weekly usage range was from a low of about 195 units toward the end of May to 395 units around January or February. Thus, our blood supplier was expected to deal with an unplanned difference of blood use of 200 units a week or almost 100 percent of the lowest weekly use.

Some of these lower usage weeks can be accounted for by certain events, but others cannot. For Memorial Day week, which is a shorter work week, there was a decrease in blood utilization. On the other hand, during the Fourth of July week and Labor Day week there was not the kind of decrease that we saw with the Memorial Day week. Christmas week is not one of our lower weeks, although Thanksgiving week did show decreased blood use. So, holidays had some effect, but not always the effect that we might have expected.

I have no explanation for the two peaks in utilization in early September and mid-January. I believe with tracking of relevant patient-related activity it would be possible to determine the causes of the increased blood use. Thus, although we often think that holiday weeks affect this balance between supply and utilization, in our experience last year they didn't affect utilization as much as we might have thought.

What are some of the reasons for these fluctuations? The week that the American College of Surgeons meets is something that we notice. When most of the surgeons are out of town, the elective surgery schedule is decreased and the blood utilization that week is lower. Short work weeks affect the elective surgery schedule, and this also is noticeable, but as we have seen, not dependably so. Medical meetings other than surgical meetings usually don't have that much of an effect on blood utilization.

Another source of variation can be one or two particular patients, such as a major trauma case, who might use 50, 60, or 70 units of red cells. A unique patient mix may also affect blood use. For instance, if one or two organ donors become available and most of those organs match patients, our hospital might do multiple transplants in the course of 24–48 hours—a couple of

BLOOD SUPPLY FLUCTUATIONS

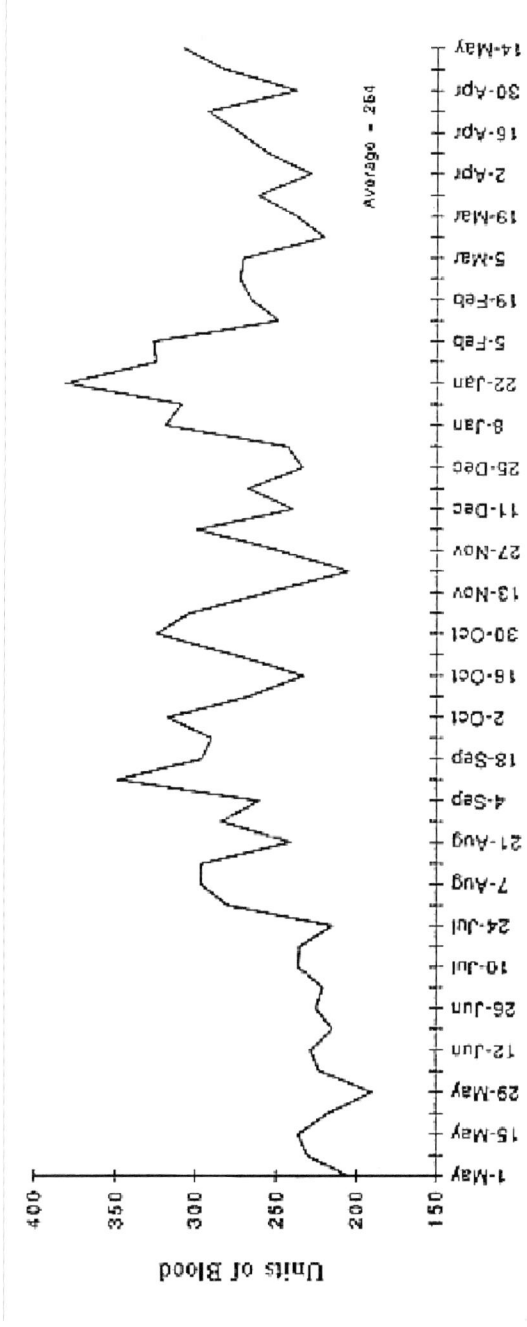

Figure 1
Weekly red blood cell use at the University of Minnesota, 1994–1995.

livers, several kidneys, and a heart. A unique set of circumstances can arise in this way in a period of a day or two and place a very substantial demand on red cells.

Another example is that sometimes groups of patients just fall together. For instance, a large bone marrow transplant program may have about 40 beds on the unit. There will be times when 10 or 12 patients may be discharged at about the same time. If you have about 12 new patients all coming on the transplant unit within a couple of days of each other, there is a huge change in the blood demands over a period of about a week because of this confluence of patient factors. Last on this list is a major disaster. This is something we talk about and think about, but, in fact, it doesn't turn out to be that much of a factor in all this because these are such rare events.

We have been discussing fluctuations in blood utilization. Now, let's consider the supply side. With supply, we have a more dependable change in blood availability. There are some periods of the year—in May, in October—when there is a substantial difference between what we actually collected and what we had planned to collect. For the most part, though, blood production coincides with the planned amount to be collected.

If these collection goals were tightly related to the projected blood needs, these time periods would be potential problems of lack of supply. The American Red Cross national data for June 1992 to April 1995 (Figure 2, kindly provided by Brian McDonough) reveals considerable monthly fluctuation. Monthly collections varied from about 440,000 to 540,000 units, a range of about 20 percent of the lowest monthly collection. If we look at the data from the North Central Region of the ARC, which includes Minnesota, we see collections averaging around 4,000 to 4,100 units a week (Figure 3). On a short week, it drops down to under 3,000, but most weeks it runs closer to 4,000. Toby Simon could show you similar data from Phoenix and Chicago, including some of the same kinds of differences between budgeted and actual collections.

Another way to consider these same data, the fluctuation in blood availability, is based on deviation from the projected blood collections. In one blood collection center, it ranged from a high of 130 percent of what they planned to collect to a low of around 75 percent of what they planned to collect, which has been our experience in St. Paul.

Many of the factors causing this fluctuation are local. One of these is the weather. It is too hot, or it is too cold. It may be that it rained, or that it didn't rain and it has been dry for two weeks. It may be that there was a blizzard. It seems as if whatever is happening out there is the reason that is used to account for why we didn't collect the blood that we thought we needed. The weather is not a common factor that affects blood availability,

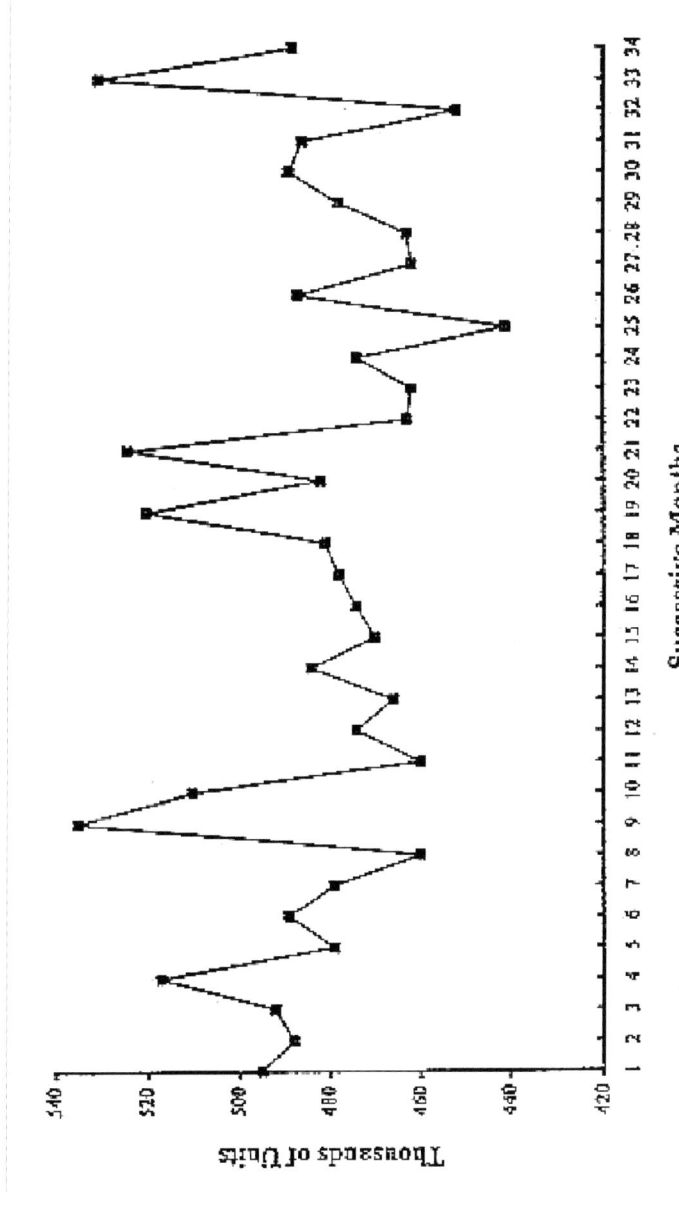

Figure 2
Monthly whole blood collections by the American Red Cross, June 1992–April 1995.

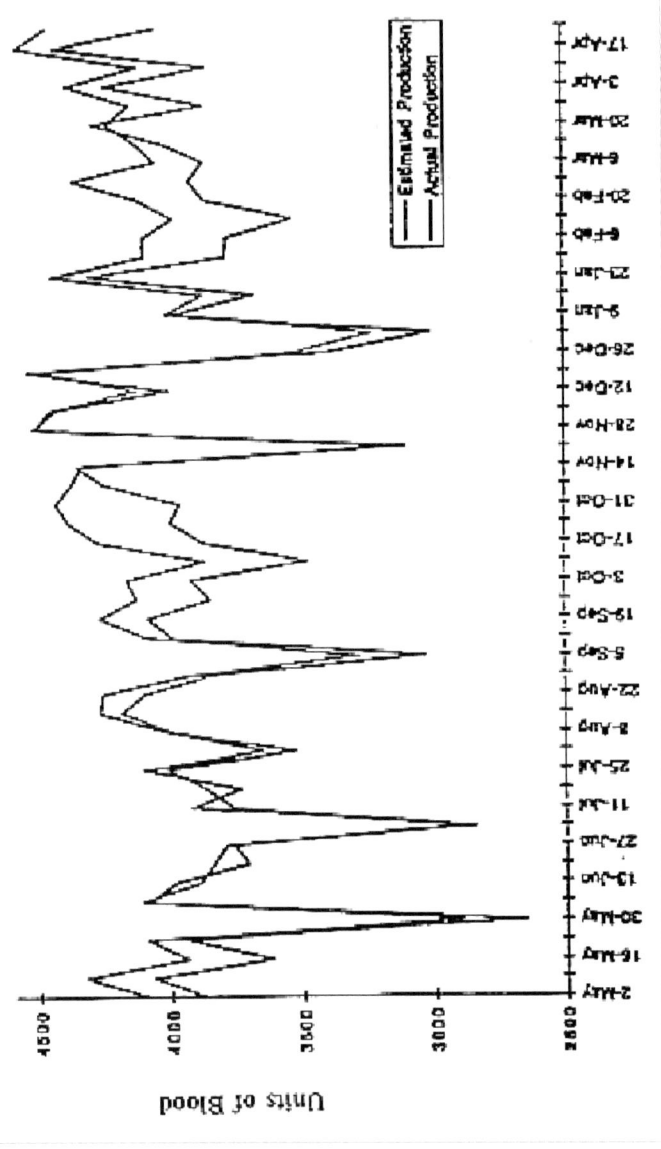

Figure 3
Estimated and actual weekly red blood cell collections by the American Red Cross North Central Region, May 1994–April 1995.

but when it does, it certainly can be a very major issue.

Time of year is another factor in blood collections. We find in general that spring is a much more effective time to operate a blood drive in high schools and colleges. High school students age during the year, so you have a larger proportion of students toward the end of the school year old enough to donate blood than in the fall.

Another consideration is work or manufacturing plant schedules, depending on how the manufacturing plant is running and whether or not they change their schedules. Probably the most important factor, however, that determines blood availability and consistency of supply is the donor recruitment staff at the blood center. A qualified, knowledgeable staff can have an enormous effect on increasing blood availability.

There are no solid answers to the issue of fluctuations in blood use and supply, partly because the factors that may influence utilization and collection are not things that we ordinarily document. Thus, we can't go back to identify at these periods of peaks and valleys what exactly was happening in the hospital to account for changes in utilization or exactly what was happening in the blood collection system to account for changes in availability. As with so many things, improved data would be valuable.

QUESTIONS/COMMENTS

Steve Bradshaw: I recently entered this area of expertise from the orthopedic business, and it was interesting to me to see the seasonality of blood usage vary with the orthopedic schedule of seasonality factors. There are over a half a million procedures of joint replacement annually, and they use as much as three to five units of blood. Seasonally, it occurs more toward the colder time of the year and ties into some of the other points you have made.

Alvin Drake: What is the rate of surgery in your hospital? Is the blood there when it is needed? Is the issue that it is difficult to get it? Or is the issue that it is not there when you need it?

Jeffrey McCullogh: We don't have a problem with blood availability. In 20 years, I can't remember being unable to do surgical procedures because of the lack of blood. The issue is more to try to match supply with demand, avoid wastage as well as shortages, and be optimally cost-effective.

Harvey Klein: But in all fairness, you are an exporter. How about some people who are importers?

Jeffrey McCullough: Yes, we are quite unusual because we collect twice as much as we use locally, and the rest of it is exported to other parts of the country.

William Sherwood: I'm with the Red Cross in Philadelphia, and we are an importer. We do have very little delay of elective surgery. Virtually all of our surgery is taken care of. There are only a very small number of cases per year where there is cancellation of elective surgery, and it is at some of those times that were pointed out. There is another practical matter. A blood center can't build in a capacity to have an enormous collection at one peak and then people sitting on their hands for a very short period of time. So, the capacity planning often limits what you can collect at any given point in time. We plan capacity for a little bit over what that median would be, so there are times that we can collect from all the donors we want to provide for and times that we have more capacity available than donors. So, capacity planning and the capacity of a blood center are as important for the short-term fluctuations as the real availability of the blood supply.

S. Gerald Sandler: From a hospital perspective, I would like to point out that the inference that it is bad to have a shortage isn't always true. When there is a shortage in Washington, for example, on platelets, we will drop the trigger for obtaining platelets from 20,000 mm^3 to 5,000 mm^3 at the hospital level and get to where we probably should be anyway. If there is a shortage of red cells, we will be forced to go back to the level we probably should use. No one has bled to death in Washington during a shortage. We have probably come closer to the levels that we should be using for our triggers.

Jeffrey McCullough: There is a related theme that I would like to mention. A friend and colleague of mine in Minneapolis, Herb Polesky, got into a fairly vigorous debate at the state medical association meeting a few years ago when he took the position that it was okay periodically to have blood shortages because it brought to the attention of the physicians that blood is not just a casual resource out there in unlimited supply. He noticed that during and shortly after blood shortages, physicians took their decisions about transfusions much more seriously and that it was actually easier to get them involved in helping to recruit blood donors.

Ronald Gilcher: A comment and a question. The comment is that it is very clear to me that if we had a steady flow of donations, it would be much better from the standpoint of staffing and not having to pay overtime at the times when you overcollect. My question is when we look at the valleys that you mentioned, they were both budgeted and actual. Was it budgeted because your recruitment staff thought that they couldn't collect or was it because you decided you didn't want to collect at that time? The reason I make that comment is we actually tend to overcollect around the holidays because our center gets requests from all over the country because of shortages, and, in fact, we do budget and we are able to overcollect at the time of the holidays.

Jeffrey McCullough: I think a lot of the things that some donor recruitment people take as givens of what they can and can't do are probably not really givens at all, and for the most part, those low weeks were planned low weeks because people thought that they couldn't get the blood.

Celso Bianco: I think that we are all beginning to realize that many of these valleys and peaks are management issues that are very difficult to deal with. I remember the *New York Times* article that was very critical of our shortages about a year or two ago. We can plan for Christmas. Christmas happens every year, and I think that we and most of the blood centers have learned how to manage. I think that we cannot plan for certain events that occur in the country. For some reason donors decide either that they want to donate a lot—and the Gulf War is a good example, along with the bombing in Oklahoma City—or they don't, and the blood supply dries up. I think that that is the part of the problem on which we have to focus. In New York we learned for instance that when we need to import, we can do that. We oscillate; in certain months, such as May and June, we will collect 30,000 units a month, but we will collect 40,000 units a month in July and August and we learn how to manage that.

Thomas Zuck: There is a corollary to the argument you and Herb had. You looked at it from the usage side. Ron Franzmeier, who most of us knew, used to say that it wasn't bad to have an appeal every now and then because the general public knows you are still there and still need blood.

Harvey Klein: I would like to ask you two questions. The first is the data that you presented were for red cells. Is there a problem with platelets as well, which clearly are different with the increase in growth of single donor platelets? Second, couldn't we totally eliminate the issue of shortages by using frozen depots in the United States? Couldn't we eliminate that problem at a cost?

Jeffrey McCullough: Platelets are a more difficult issue because of the shorter shelf life. As Bill Sherwood mentioned, with 42 days of red cells, there is a lot more latitude, whereas long weekends can be difficult for platelets. I also agree with Dr. Bianco that we are supposed to be the professionals and we are supposed to be able to plan and manage for this. I think we have allowed more excuses to be foisted on us than is probably appropriate.

Regarding frozen red cells, I suppose the answer is "Yes, it could be done if you don't care how much it costs." To try to plan for a system in which for a few days you could deglycerolize huge numbers of red cells would be very costly and inefficient. I don't think it is a practical alternative.

Paul McCurdy: Jeff, your hospital weekly utilization data were very interesting and probably not too surprising. I suspect that if you look at the same data from the standpoint of the so-called blood center you may find they don't fluctuate a great deal because when one hospital is up, another one is down. The exceptions would be smaller blood centers and places where there is one major hospital that uses almost all of the blood supply, so that their fluctuation goes to the blood center.

When Should Physicians Transfuse?

Jeffrey L. Carson

My job today is to tell you whether we in the practice of clinical medicine are appropriately using red cell transfusions. I will try to create for you a framework for a transfusion decision and what approaches have been used to determine what the appropriate use of transfusions has been. I will then show you some relevant animal data, and finally I will turn to two studies that we are in the process of completing: one we call Anemia and Surgery and the second is Surgical Blood Transfusion Variation and Outcome. I will try to convince you that we need large randomized clinical trials to answer this question definitively and that we will never know what the appropriate use is unless we get more data.

I think about transfusions in the following way. The first question I want to know is what are the mortality and morbidity levels associated with different levels of hemoglobin and how are those affected by age, comorbidity, the nature of the surgical procedure, and operative blood loss. These are issues that I think need to be incorporated into any transfusion decision. Second, if you understand what these mortality and morbidity levels are, how much can they be reduced by transfusion? Third, of course, is if you can reduce the immediate mortality and morbidity, at what risk is the patient from side effects of transfusion?

Now, this can be looked at in a slightly different way. If we were to take a surgical environment, where you are trying to make a decision to transfuse or not transfuse, and you decide to transfuse that patient, there is going to be a mortality associated with surgery that may or may not be influenced by the transfusion. The patient may survive. If the patient survives, then he or she is at risk for complications of transfusion, which include HIV, hepatitis, and perhaps bacterial infections, which may, in fact, be the most important adverse event related to transfusion.

You can add up the risks and benefits and compare them with those in the group you don't transfuse. Then you try to decide whether those who were transfused do better than those who were not transfused. And then, of course, you need to look at this in subgroups, such as those with underlying heart disease, how old they are, and the nature of the blood loss in surgical procedures. Finally, we must consider the economic consequences of transfusion decisions.

What approaches have been used to try to determine whether there is appropriate blood use? It has been mostly expert opinion. For example, the criteria for transfusion have changed during the past decade. For many years, we were using the 10–30 rule (hemoglobin below 10 g/dl and/or hematocrit below 30 percent). Then in 1988, NIH's consensus conference rejected the 10–30 rule and said that this doesn't make sense, that we ought to not be using specific hemoglobin criteria, and that we ought to be looking at other factors as well. The consensus conference suggested that perhaps 7 to 8 g/dl is a more appropriate hemoglobin level for deciding to transfuse. Of course, this is unsupported as well.

There have been several studies examining the appropriateness of transfusions. I will review one today that was published by Soumerai and colleagues[2] in 1993. In this study a group of experts from the Boston area decided on the appropriate indicators for transfusion. These included a pre-transfusion hematocrit of 24 percent and a hemoglobin of 8 g/dl; a fall of hematocrit of greater than or equal to 6 percent in those who had hematocrits between 24 and 30 percent, if they had a history of angina within 24 hours; a myocardial infarction (MI) within the past six weeks; an electrocardiogram which showed ischemic changes; or 1,000 cc of blood loss.

What they found was that about 40 percent of their transfusions were not appropriate by their criteria. About 20 to 25 percent were appropriate and the remaining were a so-called indeterminate group, with hematocrits between 24 and 30 percent, for whom they couldn't decide if the transfusion was appropriate.

They then tried to educate the doctors. They gave lectures and also met with these doctors face to face. They were able to increase somewhat the number of appropriate transfusions, up into the range of 40 percent or so, and they were able to reduce the number of inappropriate transfusions. In the control groups there was no change in the proportion of appropriate transfusions.

This study shows that after an educational program, the proportion of appropriate transfusions increases. The question remaining is whether these are truly the appropriate criteria for transfusion. I think they are quite reasonable, but I am not sure they are the best ones.

What other data are there to guide transfusion decisions? There is very

---

[2] Soumerai, SB, S Salem-Schatz, J Avorn, CS Casteris, D Ross-Degnan and MA Popovsky (1993). A controlled trial of educational outreach to improve blood transfusion practice. *Journal of the American Medical Association, 270(8)*, 961–966.

limited experimental evidence in humans to guide therapy. There have been a number of observational studies, but my view is that they are either seriously flawed or not large enough to answer this question. There has never been a randomized trial large enough to adequately evaluate blood transfusions in any clinical setting.

There are some animal data to draw upon, and if we examine how well animals tolerate anemia, what you find is that normal animals can tolerate anemia down to about about 5 g/dl. At a hemoglobin level of 5 g/dl, changes on the ST segment of the electrocardiogram begin, and below 3 g/dl, lactate production and decreased ventricular function begin and the animals begin to die.

The second point is that when coronary artery disease is experimentally induced by tying off animals' coronary arteries, reducing blood flow 50 to 70 percent, these animals are much less tolerant of anemia than normal animals. Animals with coronary obstruction develop ST segment changes at between 7 and 10 grams.

Obviously, such experiments cannot be done with humans, but I would now like to talk about two studies we are doing that ask similar questions in an ethical approximation. The first I call Anemia and Surgery. The second is a variation of a transfusion practice study. I need to emphasize that we are not done with these studies and what I am going to share with you are preliminary results.

The aims of the Anemia and Surgery study were to estimate the risk of death associated with pre- and postoperative hemoglobin levels and to determine the level of hemoglobin at which mortality begins to rise, controlling for things such as age and morbidity of surgical procedures.

We performed a retrospective cohort study of patients who refused blood transfusion for religious reasons. We were able to recruit surgeons from throughout the country who would allow us to copy their patients' charts, eliminate identifying information, and then have these medical records reviewed by nurse abstractors. We collected information on demographics, comorbidity, and preop hemoglobin levels. Our main outcome measure was 30-day mortality, which was assessed by medical record review and the National Death Index (NDI) Search.

For patients to be eligible for our study, we required evidence in the medical record that the patient would refuse blood transfusion if offered and that the patient underwent a surgical procedure in the operating room. We excluded open heart cases because of the nature of the procedure and blood use there, and we required a preop hemoglobin level in their chart. We restricted the study to those 18 years of age or older because the courts could have forced younger Jehovah's Witnesses to take blood. We had a total of 2,102 patients, of which 1,958 were ages 18 or older. I want to emphasize one point, which is that we have a variable that we call cardiovascular disease, which includes a history of MI, angina, congestive heart failure, or a history of peripheral vascular disease.

What were some of our results? In this group of 1,958 patients, only 3.2 percent died. We have concluded from this preliminary analysis that surgical mortality was very low in this population who declined blood transfusion, and that it increases with declining hemoglobin levels in patients with cardiovascular disease. In patients with a preoperative hemoglobin of 10 or less, mortality is much more sensitive to preop hemoglobin in patients with cardiovascular disease than in those without such disease. These results suggest that the hemoglobin trigger for transfusion should be at a higher level in patients with cardiac disease than in those without cardiac disease. However, I think a randomized trial is needed to establish whatever the transfusion trigger should be.

We are not nearly as far along on the second study I am going to tell you about. This is a study called Surgical Blood Transfusion Variation and Outcome. It is funded by the Agency for Health Care Policy and Research (AHCPR), and the aims of this particular study are to understand the independent predictors of transfusion practices. We will determine if surgeons are transfusing for comorbidity, age, or other patient characteristics or whether they are using a transfusion trigger. The second aim of the study is to describe the effect of transfusion on postoperative mortality and morbidity. We will study these questions in cases of hip fractures undergoing surgical repair, using 30-day mortality as our primary outcome. Secondary outcomes include mortality up to one year, in-hospital morbidity, bacterial infections, length of stay, and disposition as well as some very simple functional status measures.

The study will include 10,000 hip fracture patients, from four geographic regions, who underwent surgery during the past ten years. So far, we have only collected the data. We are about two weeks away from having our mortality data all defined. It is probably not going to be until the end of the summer that I have some good preliminary results. What we plan to do is to describe the mortality and morbidity in patients who are transfused compared to those in patients who are not transfused.

How do these studies all fit together? How do they try to get at the answer to this question of who we should be transfusing? I think the Anemia and Surgery study identifies the hemoglobin levels at which the death rate begins to rise, above which you clearly wouldn't consider transfusing. However, it doesn't tell you whether transfusion is going to impact that increased mortality we were seeing. We expect that the variation study will evaluate the effect of blood transfusion on this death rate and how at different hemoglobin levels transfusion affects postoperative mortality and morbidity.

Both of these studies are observational, however, and we will never know for sure if we completely control for confounding variables. Therefore, a randomized trial will absolutely be needed to define the transfusion trigger. The basic idea of such a study is to contrast two transfusion triggers. I am waiting to see what our observational studies show before we decide what these comparison groups should be. We are proposing to do a very large simple randomized clinical trial in hip fracture patients using 30-day mortality as our primary outcome. The real unknown at this point is the number of patients that we need in this trial. Until I finish the hip fracture study and get my 30-day mortality data, I can't do my sample size calculations.

I would summarize my formal remarks by saying we currently have very few data to guide transfusion decisions. One observational study suggests that patients with cardiovascular disease should be transfused at a higher hemoglobin level than those without cardiovascular disease. However, additional data are required to determine who truly should be transfused, and I think a randomized trial is clearly needed. Without such data, it is very hard for me to answer the question of whether red cells are being appropriately used. My answer is that I don't know. I think there is evidence to suggest that maybe they are not, but I think until you can provide doctors with clear evidence about what they should and shouldn't do, it is hard to convince them that they are doing things inappropriately.

QUESTIONS/COMMENTS

Eve Lackritz: What proportion of blood is being used in the surgical setting?

Jeffrey Carson: My sense is that it is probably 80 percent.

Douglas Surgenor: I don't think anybody has a firm number in a large sense.

Jeffrey Carson: I suspect the blood centers have a sense that it is most of the blood supply. It is certainly well over 50 percent.

William Sherwood: Mortality is a nice, clean end point. I am wondering if there are other parameters, though, that are useful to evaluate.

Jeffrey Carson: I couldn't agree more with you. I would be pleased to talk to you later about the problems in trying to do a study of this sort. The basic problem is that with mortality outcome, you don't need the blinded trial. Think about how you might try to blind doctor and patient to who is getting a unit of blood. I think you can't do that practically. You could blind hemoglobin levels to the physicians and the patients and so still keep their assigned groups blinded. The practical part of that is that it is going to require more money to pull that off.

Let's create a scenario in which you show no difference in mortality and morbidity, you show no difference in functional status, but you show a prolonged length of stay or perhaps that more of these older folks are going to nursing homes if they don't get transfused. If I showed that one variable that was significant and nothing else, that would be almost enough reason for me to consider transfusing someone.

I absolutely agree with you that those secondary outcomes would be very important to include in your analysis. It is an issue of how you can do this when you have morbidity as the outcome, which in principle is subject to bias. It is harder to do, but I don't believe that it is an unsurmountable problem.

C. Robert Valeri: The issue that you should look at is whether or not the hemoglobin concentration per se has an important impact on hemostasis.

Jeffrey Carson: They are correlated. Those who bleed have lower hemoglobins. How do you dissect that out? I don't think you can dissect that.

C. Robert Valeri: There are good data to suggest that with anemia, you produce platelet dysfunction. If you are very anemic, you may make the platelets dysfunction, and therefore, you are going to bleed more. So, it would be important to consider surgical patients who are bleeding to be in need of transfused red cells, regardless of their hemoglobin level, to help platelet function.

Harvey Klein: I think one of the points we wanted to make here is that we all assume that too much blood is being transfused in the United States, and it is clear that we really don't know that for certain. In some instances it may be that too little is being transfused.

International Perspectives on Blood Availability

Robert G. Westphal

I've been asked to talk to you today about the international perspective because I just returned from spending three years in Geneva, Switzerland as a Medical Advisor in the Blood Programme Department of the International Federation of Red Cross and Red Crescent Societies. However, I didn't spend much time in Geneva looking at Western European blood programs. I spent a lot of time looking at developing programs, so I don't consider myself an expert on blood transfusion in Western Europe. However, I do have some items I think we can focus on and possibly learn from.

Comparing Europe with the United States, I think that we in the United States have some problems with the way we handle our donors and consequently with getting our donors back. To put it a different way, I think we have reagent problems in our blood industry.

It wasn't until the end of the 1980s that we began to actually regulate blood component production as a drug manufacturing process. We have overdone it a bit, and it is not entirely the fault of the regulatory agencies. When the regulatory agencies said to build a 12-foot wall, in many cases we built a 20-foot wall. We actually now have a category of "biohazardous donors" whom we treat in an absurdly onerous fashion.

Our donors are the only reagents I know of that change their shape. They forget their birthdays and other identifying numbers. They change their names. They move. They have conjugal relationships with other reagents. They are just not reagents in the classical sense. We should take another look at how we treat them and develop a different view of them.

There is a totally unreported infectious disease that is present in our blood programs today and that is a transfusion-related infection I call the bipolar AA virus. I think we create so much anger and so much apathy—and that is why it is bipolar—in our donors that we are having a lot of trouble. A lot of these remarks are really directed to the panels that will be coming up to discuss some of these issues. We spread this virus fairly readily, and I think we need to look at how we are treating our donors if we want them to keep coming back. I think the compounding of autologous and directed collections in this has not helped us.

What are some of the causes of this AA virus infection? Most of you could promulgate a list as easily as I could. First, we have a tremendous number of donors who are deferred for unnecessary reasons. The American Red Cross alone defers 1.2 million donors per year because of elevated liver enzymes (ALT), mostly false positives. In the Northeast Region in two states, Massachusetts and Maine, after hepatitis C virus (HCV) tests became available in 1990, we lost about 20,000 donors to generally falsely positive ALT tests. To that can be added roughly the same number from false-positive hepatitis B core antibody tests and 3,000 nonconfirmed HIV-positive tests. This is not an insignificant number of donors. Furthermore, they have friends and their friends look at these letters that they get and they are quite concerned.

We also have what Merlyn Sayers described as the donor interrogation or donor inquisition, as some of us have come to call it. I am sure that all of you have seen this letter from a donor in the *CCBC Newsletter* . I will read some of it in case you haven't seen it.

This is from a 66-year-old man, who has given 11 gallons of blood. He wrote, "Thirty years ago, I got in the habit of donating blood regularly, averaging three times a year. Unfortunately, in recent years, my blood center has made the process so ugly and repugnant, that I have quit. In the case of my blood center, protecting the regulators and the blood center against lawsuits has displaced gathering blood as the primary function. At the predonation interview, a nurse young enough to be my granddaughter asked me a massive series of ugly questions, including those I wouldn't discuss with my male friends. At the end she tells me she knows there is still a good chance that I might have lied in answering all those questions, so she is going to give me one last chance to not withhold the truth. She will give me a moment of privacy where I can relent and fix the bar code warning that I did, in fact, lie."

"Wouldn't it be reasonable to expect that after 30 years of testing and transfusing my blood, over and over again verifying that it is clean and safe, that the blood center's computer system would know that, know me, trust me, and want me? I should have an ID card with a magnetic strip they could run through a reader. After verification of my identity, the question they should ask is, 'Any change since the last time?' If 'No,' skip the next 100 grossly intrusive questions."

He continues in this vein and as a caveat, he says, "I am sure you are thinking that I am just a grumpy old man, but ask yourself how many other grumpy old men and women have stopped coming to give blood to you for those reasons."

He makes two points. One is about the donor interrogation, and the other is that confidential unit exclusion is ambiguous for donors because on the one hand, they are all expected to tell the truth, but some of them can lie if they want and then check another box. We have learned that it is not a very satisfactory means, at least these days, in most centers for us to screen donors.

There are many examples of the confusing, vague, and frightening letters we send to donors. The country's largest blood collector has now abandoned the whole idea of reentering donors who have false-positive tests. We are also proposing questions to eliminate donors who might be at risk for a very unusual illness, Creutzfeldt-Jakob disease (CJD), caused by something we have not completely identified and cannot confidently say is infectious in the blood transfusion sense. To ask donors questions to prevent something with which they might become infected in the future, or may have in their family but don't know about, is quite a leap into chaos.

Many countries don't do direct questioning of donors. Many countries don't do some of the tests we do, and therefore, they don't have some of the results that we do. For example, ALT testing, HBV core testing, and HTLV-1 and -2 testing are not done in most of the major European countries. The Europeans have also made the absolutely marvelous discovery that the best place to store blood is in the human body. They do very little autologous collection, and they do virtually no directed donations. And the reason they don't is because the patients believe their doctors who tell them that it is not always needed (autologous) and that it is not safer blood (directed).

Major shipments come from several countries in Europe to a well-known blood center in the United States. It is a very good idea. I used to be in a region where we had the opportunity to collect an excess amount of blood and ship it to other regional centers. We were able to help regions that had some shortages. However, when you ship competitively to *hospitals*, it is disruptive to planning and meeting needs. Then the costs of providing services tend to go up within that region. This doesn't happen in Europe. There are shipments between national blood program centers to other national blood program centers and just a few shipments from one country to another, but really very little of that.

Let me share with you some numbers from the Council of Europe for the year 1989. That same year in Japan and the United States the collections per 1,000 population were 65 and 54, respectively. In Belgium, Denmark, France, to some degree in Luxembourg, and to a tremendous degree in Switzerland, there was a much greater rate of donation. The numbers on Eastern Europe for 1992 get worse. From 1992 to 1993, these have gone down in countries such as Albania, Bulgaria, Romania, and Czech Republic. You see massive declines in the number of blood donations there (See Table 2).

TABLE 2 Number of Voluntary, Nonremunerated Blood Donations per 1,000 Inhabitants in 1989, by European Country

Country	Donations/1,000	Country	Donations/1,000
Albania	44	Lithuania	35
Belgium	68	Luxembourg	56
Bulgaria	24	Netherlands	52
Czech Republic	36	Poland	23
Denmark	83	Portugal	18
Estonia	51	Romania	26
France	70	Slovakia	31
Germany	44	Slovenia	51
Greece	42	Spain	25
Hungary	47	Switzerland	100
Ireland	37	United Kingdom	44
Italy	31		

But the real question is why are some of these countries in Western Europe doing so well? How can they collect so much blood? I don't know what the answer is exactly. I can tell you that after talking with several people over there, I have a somewhat different picture of the blood recruitment and collection process than what we have in the United States.

First of all, in general, the collection and/or public education responsibility in Western European countries is given to a single authority in the country, generally under the auspices of some kind of national blood program and policy. Another major difference is that the people responsible for collection and/or donor recruitment invest a major effort at the very highest levels to meet with their counterparts in other organizations and get the recruitment message out to the public. In the United States, this work tends to devolve down to a fairly low common denominator of a donor recruitment person going out and talking with someone at their level at a plant or company, school, or college or university.

There aren't enough big shots involved in donor recruitment in the United States compared to Europe. In Europe there is a great deal of effort, much of which goes back through the history of World War II, to make the program a part of each community. Each community, then, has a real commitment to themselves to provide for their blood needs. In Switzerland, for example, there is a group of almost paramilitary, paramedical personnel, with traditions dating back to World War II, who have a membership of about a million. These million people are one-seventh of the population of Switzerland, and they comprise a major recruitment group. They go out and run blood drives and they do it at a very grassroots level. Sometimes they do it at a somewhat socially coercive level, but it is very effective.

In Europe, many cities have a sense of community, which I think we lack in many of the cities in the United States. We are just too big. Our messages get totally diluted because of the size and because there are so many other things that are going on. It is a little bit like the rural ethic and the urban ethic. If you live in the country, people know if they don't take care of it, it won't get done, whereas in the larger areas, people think someone else is going to do it.

The other thing in Europe is they don't talk so much about donor recruitment. They talk about donor retention. They want to get their old donors back, the ones that they know, who are safer and easier to find. This donor retention is a multidisciplinary effort, and they all work at it, from the top guy in the Swiss Red Cross right on down.

In addition, young people are viewed in Europe as the key to the future of blood transfusion. Blood needs are part of the biology curriculum in some European schools. The blood service operates as a public trust, and the public expects a tremendous amount of accountability. They ask for it and they generally get it.

So, in summary, in comparing my long experience in the States with my brief experience in Europe, one of the biggest differences has to do with how we treat our donors. Generally speaking, in Europe the donors are treated much more charitably and much more gratefully. In the United States, the donor is viewed with suspicion. He is lying. Otherwise, we would have no confidential unit exclusion (CUE). Donors who have positive infectious disease results that are confirmed positives are generally not notified by letter in Europe. They receive an invitation to visit the doctor, their own or the blood center's. In the United States, they are judged, sentenced, and practically put away by mail with some of these awful letters that all of you know about.

There is much more local autonomy, not so much in regulated areas but in how you organize a blood drive, how you set it up, the rules for collecting and who can be a donor, and what the minimum standards should be. These are not the very precisely defined standards that some of us try to spread across the country, which can be very difficult because communities are different and they expect different things.

Most Europeans don't do direct questioning of donors. They give them the form. They review it carefully. If they have questions about it later, they may call them or if the form isn't filled out right, they will go back to them, but they don't do the donor inquisition. The European forms are simpler in general, but most of the forms look very much like ours. The questions asked in the countries that export blood to the United States, obviously, include all of the questions that we ask in the United States. They don't do much CUE, and in general, their donors are valued and honored more than ours are.

Jim Mosley noted in 1991 in an article in *Transfusion*: "The intricacy and complexity which one can get into can overwhelm an honest donor and overwhelm a conscientious interviewer."[3] We have exceeded the limits of sensitivity and specificity of the donor questionnaire in excluding hazardous donations. What we are doing to our donors is really unconscionable. I think it is one of the reasons we have trouble with our blood supply. People are saving it up. They don't want the hassle. They will give their own blood when they need it. If a friend asks them to give, maybe they will. And I think that something can be done about that.

QUESTIONS/COMMENTS

Arthur Caplan: One of the things you said near the end of your talk was that public accountability is important. I spent the past two days thinking about Mickey Mantle because the public these days is very concerned about issues of equity and fairness in the distribution of organs. One of the issues that comes up with respect to Mr. Mantle and his liver transplant is whether or not the distribution system that is out there is fair and equitable. We have some recent studies that point directly to distrust and mistrust of the system's distribution patterns as reasons for people not to participate in organ donation and tissue donation. This is particularly true for poor and minority people, who basically look at the system and say, "If I can't benefit, I won't donate to it and I won't carry a card and I am not going to be interested in what happens with respect to making my organs or tissues available upon my death."

That is a lesson that may or may not carry into the blood world as well. I know it is true in the organ and tissue world. It comes up with people who either are celebrities or have the ability to command resources out of the system that others can't. Thus, I offer the speakers on the next panel the hypothesis that accountability with respect to distribution and allocation of resources is crucial to understanding how to enhance and find ways to encourage both donor participation and donor retention.

---

[3] Mosley, JW (1991). Who should be our blood donors? *Transfusion, 31:* 684–685.

II
ENHANCING COLLECTIONS

The Delaware Plan

David Bonk

I am here to tell you about the unique system of blood procurement, called the Delaware Plan, that has been developed in my area of the country. In the way of background, you should know that the Blood Bank of Delaware is a medium-sized blood bank, serving 19 hospitals on the Delmarva Peninsula, which includes the state of Delaware and the Eastern Shore of Maryland. We annually draw about 55,000 units of whole blood and platelet apheresis products and distribute approximately 90,000 units of blood and blood products to those 19 hospitals. We are very proud of the fact that in over 30 years we have not had a blood shortage or a cancelled surgery for lack of blood, or an emergency appeal for blood donors. Hospitals in our area set their own optimal inventory levels. They get whatever they want whenever they ask for it. Compared to the national strategy of having donors give three to four times per year, we ask our members to take a turn approximately once every two years.

Of the one million residents in our area, nearly 700,000 are covered by our membership plan. Compared to the national average of 3 to 5 percent of the eligible population giving blood, in our area 20 to 25 percent of the eligible population gives blood. We don't conduct community blood drives. We never hold blood drives at businesses.

Anytime more blood is needed, even Type O, that need can be met quickly and without alarm or additional cost. We have a blood program that works very effectively at the one thing that blood banks are supposed to do and that is provide a reliable supply of high-quality blood products to the hospitals we serve every day of the year, no exceptions, no excuses.

We also have the lowest processing fees in our area of the country, and the savings to those hospitals in terms of lower fees, reliable supplies, and the elimination of cancelled surgeries for lack of blood have been enormous. All of this has been accomplished through our membership blood assurance plan, the Delaware Plan. It is an unusual way for a blood bank to function, so I will tell you a little bit about the way it works.

We ask people to join our membership plan as a means of providing blood for the community and coverage for themselves and their families. Each membership is a family plan, providing coverage for the member, the member's spouse, and all tax dependents. Each member family is asked to do two things. First, we ask them to pay a small annual dues to keep the membership active. That is either $2 or $5, depending on age. Second, we ask them to provide a pint of blood when it is their turn. In return, people who join and support our program pay reduced fees when they or their family members use blood. This is a credit system. The 19 hospitals we serve charge a replacement deposit fee (RDF) for the patients who use blood and are not members of the blood bank's plan. This fee, which is $30 for a unit of red cells and $15 for a unit of platelets, could be paid or the charges waived if the blood is replaced.

For example, if a nonmember uses 10 units of packed cells, the processing fee at $57.50 per unit would total $575. The replacement deposit fee at $30 per unit would total $300. The total bill for this patient, who is not a blood bank member, would thus be $875. Generally, health insurance does not pay the RDF. That same patient as a blood bank member would be charged the processing fee at $57.50 per unit, but would not be charged the replacement fee for a total bill of $575, or a savings for that member of $300.

That is the incentive for people in our area to join and support our program, and that is why the majority of the population has joined. In exchange for this coverage, they are asked to take a turn providing an acceptable pint of blood. Since we have such a large membership base, that turn is infrequent, approximately once every two years. When it is a member's turn to provide a pint of blood, he or she has three options: either give blood himself, if eligible; provide an eligible substitute donor; or pay the $30 fee to replace one unit of blood. For those members who cannot fulfill any of those options, we provide a donation credit from a high school donor. We don't want to lose a member because they can't donate, don't know someone to donate for them, or cannot afford to pay that fee. Of course, our overall marketing goal is to make sure that everyone in our region is covered.

The key to our success is the support of businesses and organizations. As I mentioned earlier, we do not conduct community blood drives and we don't ask businesses to sponsor blood drives. This is expensive for businesses in terms of lost worker time and productivity. We simply ask businesses and organizations to be group sponsors of our membership plan. Currently, there are over 2,700 businesses, corporations, and organizations on the Delmarva Peninsula that are group sponsors with us.

Their responsibility as group sponsors is to do three things: first, recruit new members into our blood bank plan; second, provide member addresses and telephone numbers; and third, collect the $5 or $2 annual dues for each group member. Most of our groups gladly pay those dues as a fringe benefit of employment. We deal directly with the member when it is that member's time to give blood, and he or she can donate during nonworking hours on evenings or weekends. We estimate the annual cost to a business at under $10 per blood bank member. This compares with the estimated cost for a business to conduct a blood drive at somewhere between $20 and $50 per donor in lost worker time and productivity.

Between 80 and 85 percent of the blood drawn in the United States is drawn at places of business or at organizations such as churches or clubs. The remainder is drawn at fixed sites. In our plan, 94 percent of the blood is drawn at fixed sites. None is drawn at businesses. This keeps our costs down and significantly reduces the cost for each business. It encourages businesses to support our plan by recruiting members for us. Currently, we have over 182,000 members, and those memberships provide coverage for nearly 700,000 people. We are actively working to recruit the nonmembers.

Another significant difference in our area is that we are able to prescreen 95 percent of the donors before they ever come into our donor centers. When it is a member's turn to give blood, we contact him or her at home with a postal notice that contains a list of options and some of the information about who generally qualifies as a blood donor and who generally is disqualified. We include a list of the high-risk behaviors for AIDS, so that they have time to read it at home, not sitting in our waiting room.

We ask members to call to make an appointment if they plan to give blood. When they call, we are able to prescreen them over the telephone to eliminate those who would obviously not qualify. It saves a tremendous amount of time for them, which they appreciate, and it also saves time for us.

That is how the Delaware Plan works. It is based on individual responsibility. This is an extremely equitable system in that every person is asked to play a small role in ensuring the community's blood supply. We spread that responsibility over a larger base than is common among most blood programs. Those who choose to not participate are asked to pay for or replace any blood that they use.

The system has been working extremely well, but it is not without problems. One of our biggest problems is that our members are asked to donate when it is their turn, which results in a random supply of blood types donated each day. Because we have a greater need for Type O generally, and other types from time to time, we created our Lifesaver Club. It is for people who want to donate more often than every two years. Over 12,000 of our members have joined and have agreed to be on call should we have an extra need for their type of blood. We can project that need several days in advance, and when we expect our in-house inventory to go below optimal levels, we will call and ask those next on the Lifesaver Club list if they can come in during the next few days so that we can avoid having an emergency. The donor receives an extra credit that can be used at a later date or given to a friend or relative. That system provides for nearly all of our type-specific needs.

Another concern that has come up in national forums is the safety of the blood from replacement donors compared to that from the general population of donors. In recent years, the practice of using the RDF has been under increased scrutiny. Consequently, we conducted a study to see if replacement donors are less safe than the general population of blood donors.

The results were presented at the AABB annual meeting last year. We did a comparison of test marker rates between member donors and replacement donors, to see if replacement donors had a higher incidence of test marker rate. The major hurdle was that in our system, since the majority of the population is covered and participates by donating, there are relatively few actual replacement donations. We had to review the records for two full years of donations to achieve a statistically significant sample size.

TABLE 3 Comparison of Viral Markers in Blood of Delaware Plan Members and Replacement Donors

Marker	Number (%) Member Donors (N = 67,338)	Number (%) Replacements (N = 1,354)
Hepatitis B core antibody	660 (1.0)	19 (1.4)
Hepatitis C antibody	457 (0.7)	12 (0.9)
Alanine aminotransferase	875 (1.3)	23 (1.7)
Syphilis (STS)	5 (0.01)	0
HIV-1 antibody	9 (0.01)	0
HIV-2 antibody	0	0
Hepatitis B surface antigen	4 (0.01)	0
Human T-cell lymphotropic virus antibody	4 (0.01)	0

The database was the test results from all blood donations made during the years 1992 and 1993 at our donor centers. Chi-square analysis was used to compare the repeatedly positive test results in the two groups with p greater than 0.05. Of the eight screening tests we were performing at that time, only ALT, HBcAB, and anti-HCV occurred at sufficient frequencies to be meaningfully analyzed. The difference in the incidence rate among the replacement donors compared to that among allogeneic donors was not found to be statistically significant. The study did show that replacement donors were more likely to be giving blood for the first time, 18.5 percent, and their test marker rates were similar to those of other first-time donors. Our results indicated that the blood given by replacement donors is statistically as safe as that given by the general population of donors.

The next question that often comes up when other blood bankers look at our system is whether it is fair. The replacement fee has been called a penalty fee, while others say we use the fee to coerce people to give blood. This is not how we administer the program.

As I have noted, we have less than 2 percent replacement donors, and there are ways around the fee. For example, we actively recruit ongoing blood users, so that they will be covered. Someone who is added to one of our group accounts will be covered immediately, even if he or she uses blood that same day. We have group accounts with the local heart association and the cancer society that will accept as a member anyone who is affected by heart disease or cancer.

We also discount our replacement fees to the hospitals by their annual bad debt ratio so that the hospital will not try to collect from the poor and the indigent. For example, if Hospital A has a bad debt ratio of 10 percent, we reduce the amount of the replacement fees that we charge that hospital by 10 percent. For those who cannot afford to pay our membership fee or cannot fulfill the obligation to provide blood when it is their turn, we have programs to provide free memberships or student donations for those people. I submit to you that the Delaware Plan is one of the most equitable in the nation, and I ask the following questions for the Forum to consider:

- Is it fair that 95 out of every 100 people in the United States who could give blood do not?
- Is it fair to overdraw in some areas of the country to subsidize blood programs that cannot provide for their local needs because they can't motivate their local population?
- Is it fair to the people who give blood four times a year that they receive no advantage over those who never give blood?
- Finally, is it safe to have a predictable major shortage of blood every January, every July, and every September and not attempt to change the system?

To summarize, for over 30 years, the Delaware Plan has eliminated blood shortages, eliminated surgeries cancelled for lack of blood, and eliminated emergency media appeals for blood donors. Hospitals in our system set their own optimal inventory levels for blood. People in our area are asked to give blood every two years instead of three to four times every year. Of the eligible population, 20 to 25 percent give blood under this plan, compared to 3 to 5 percent nationally. The costs to business sponsors and to our hospitals is significantly lower than those in other areas. Spreading the burden for the blood supply over a large population through this blood assurance plan is more equitable for all. It reduces the costs and provides for a steady predictable supply of blood without compromising safety. That is the Delaware Plan, and that is our approach to it.

QUESTIONS/COMMENTS

Alvin Drake: I question those statistics gravely. For reasons I will talk about, 3.5 percent of the U.S. population gives blood every year. If 25 percent of the people in Delaware gave blood in the same time period, you wouldn't know what to do with the blood. It is measured over different time periods.

David Bonk: You are correct, but we are talking about the number of people who actually participate as blood donors in our system.

Arthur Bracey: There is a notion that there are a number of people in the population that are at risk for having infectious diseases. What do you think is the desirable level of participation? What is the index for donation or participation in the donor program?

David Bonk: For our donor program, we make a great distinction between the people who we want as members and the people we want as donors. We want everyone to join and support the program in some way or other. We certainly don't want anyone who is at risk for any of the diseases to donate blood, and we are very careful with that. Our test marker rate overall in our donor population is lower than that in the other areas of our region. We are making that distinction, but our approach is to try to recruit everyone in our area to support the program in one way or another. This is not necessarily through their donation of blood, because, clearly, a lot of people don't qualify to donate and we don't want them, but we do want their support.

Thomas Zuck: How do you recruit platelet apheresis donors?

David Bonk: We do that more traditionally. Our apheresis program is separate from our membership plan. There is certainly no requirement to participate. It is more in the line of altruism, although our platelet apheresis donors do receive two credits when they make donations. We generally just recruit them by mail from among our regular blood donors or recruit them in the chair as they are giving their allogeneic unit of blood.

Ana Chinoda: In Florida, there is an outside firm which has visited all of the hospitals and has spoken with them on the diagnosis related group (DRG) reimbursement issue, showing hospitals why they should move away from the replacement deposit fee because of the three-unit deductible in Medicare. Have you not run into that problem at all in Delaware?

David Bonk: The question comes up periodically, but the system works extremely well at recruiting blood donors and maintaining one thing that we absolutely need, enough blood on the shelves every day of the year. You saw the fluctuations in some of the presentations made earlier, the highs and the lows. We don't experience any of those lows, and our outdate ratio is very low as well. The question of the replacement deposit fee almost becomes moot as you approach the level of the population that is covered that we have.

Celso Bianco: How do you deal with specific high-risk populations, for instance, gay men or with minorities? How do they have access to this plan?

David Bonk: We recruit them as members the same way we recruit any other member, and, of course, when the questions come up, we very clearly tell them that there are extensive restrictions as to who can actually donate a pint of blood, but we welcome everybody regardless of medical condition to be a member and support the program in one way or another.

William Sherwood: We have admired the success that you have had and have benefited from it. I wonder if you have given thought to how that kind of system would work in large cities, such as New York, Chicago, Philadelphia, and Los Angeles, where there are large, inner city populations. These are people who are very difficult to contact and as a group have extremely high blood usage. Do you think this could work in those kinds of environments?

David Bonk: We have thought about it, and the question has come up many times. We don't have an example of how this system would work in a large metropolitan area. We would certainly like to see if the numbers would lend themselves to trying this plan in an inner city situation, although it is impossible to say.

Markets and the Blood Supply

Lloyd Cohen

I was initially very surprised to be invited to speak here, but when I found out that Art Caplan was responsible for inviting me, I knew why I had been invited and what I was expected to say. He and I are on opposite sides of a debate having to do with organ transplants. I favor markets. To some people, I may even seem like a caricature of an economist, who, as the famous old saying goes, knows the price of everything and the value of nothing.

The position that I will assert here is the extraordinarily unexciting position that if something is valuable, the best, most efficient way of acquiring it is to pay for it. That is my view with regard to ambulances, scalpels, operating rooms, bread, housing, and clothing. There are exceptions to the general principle that simple markets in which one pays for the goods in question are the most efficient. Let me suggest three possible kinds of exceptions that might come to mind in the case of blood banking. I will dismiss two of them and then discuss the third a little bit more.

The first is a kind of general moral exception, that somehow it is elevating of the spirit that people give blood and that this all is part of the great donative act, which draws us together as a community. I think that is largely nonsense. First of all, I suspect that the people in this room think they do valuable things for other human beings and don't feel any less that way because they earn a living doing so. So, too, with providing blood to others. I don't think in any important way the act is morally elevated by not paying people rather than by paying them. Certainly not to the extent that we should prohibit, prevent, or discourage people from selling it. Beyond that, if any sacrifice to the health of innocents is entailed by our insistence on somehow keeping this a donative procedure rather than paying people, then it is truly bizarrely immoral; that is to say, if we are condemning people to mortality and morbidity, there is certainly nothing moral in doing that on the altar of encouraging the great charitable, altruistic act of donation.

The second possible exception to markets is cost. Some people may think that donation is a less costly system than paying people. It may seem odd to you, but, in fact, donation is a more costly system than paying people. Now, the illusion is that it is more costly if you have to pay money to those who sell blood. Well, indeed, it is more costly to you who must pay, but if we are looking at this from a social perspective, there is no such thing as a free lunch. Someone is gaining from the price you must pay, and someone is paying when you get the blood for free. From society's perspective, the person who is donating rather than being paid is suffering a cost.

If we count his costs as part of the whole social mix, then the fact that you haven't paid him is no cost saving at all. It is simply a transfer. This is dedicated to the proposition that there is no such thing as a free lunch, but there, indeed, are lunches that other people pay for. You are concerned with "your cost," but from a social perspective, the money that you pay for blood is not a true cost. It is just a transfer of money. The true cost is the cost of the donors who suffer discomfort, lost time, lost earnings, and travel expenses. Those are true costs. The dollar valuation of those costs is merely a measure of the value of those sacrifices of time, comfort, and resources.

From a wider perspective, donation is more costly than sale. How is it more costly? Precisely because you don't pay people in cash you frequently must compensate them in a more inefficient manner if you are going to compensate and encourage them at all. Another notion is that if you collect through blood drives at work, you are taking away time from work. It used to be the case that employers would give half a day off from work. Again, this is a payment in kind, more costly than it would be to simply pay people in cash, at a much lesser amount, to induce them to sell their blood. So, from a variety of perspectives, donations are a more costly means of acquiring blood than paying people in one form or another.

The final issue is that of monitoring. I am going to give you examples, having nothing to do with blood, to show you the generality of this problem—a number of areas in which it is difficult or impossible to pay someone for what you want because you can't measure whether you have received it or not. You can't measure it directly when you are getting it. You may not be able to measure it later. Sometimes, even if you can measure it later, the measurement comes too late to be helpful.

So, you must either supplement a simple cash market or substitute something else. So, for example, you throw in bonuses, retirement plans, and stock options as a supplement to simple wages or salary. The hope is that in this way one can induce employees to be productive when you can't measure productivity directly. The general rule is you can't get precisely what you want if you can't measure and reward precisely what you want.

Another interesting illustration I came across the other day is of a man who owns supermarkets in Northern California, in low-income areas. He needs to hire reliable employees. Some people are honest, some are dishonest, and he has a real problem sorting. It does him little good to ask them if they are honest. We have a similar problem with blood. It is not all that useful to ask people if they are HIV positive. So, what do you do?

To the extent that we have this problem that we cannot very well directly measure and monitor the safety of blood, we want to sort the population in such a way that we don't get blood from high-risk groups. We also don't want to encourage people to lie about whether or not they fall within this high-risk group.

The supposition was made that when you pay people for blood, you suffer from both of those problems: you attract people from a population more prone to falling into this high-risk category and that for that population and for other populations in general, you encourage people to be deceitful in revealing whether or not their blood is hazardous.

Now, under those circumstances, if one could find a means of getting the blood, other than paying for it, then one should give some weight to that. First, let me separate out the lying problem and the sorting problem. The lying problem is not all that much a function of whether you are paying people; that is, there is as much an incentive for people to lie if they are under peer pressure of one sort or another.

So, it is not clear that paying people for blood, particularly if we are talking about amounts of $20 or $30 per pint, is a crucial factor in whether they will conceal a health problem. If I am wrong, though, that is a point in favor of not paying for blood.

As for the sorting problem, that is an entirely separate problem. If we are trying to sort people because we don't want derelicts and we don't want gay men, that is a problem that exists independent of whether we pay people or don't pay people. I suspect that in North Dakota and in Minnesota there are fewer people who are HIV positive or have hepatitis and, so, those end up being rather safer sources for the blood supply.

This leads to a particular advantage of markets. The general pattern in the United States has been to encourage widespread donation, again, part of this whole donative ethic. From the perspective of trying to get a safe, secure, reliable, continuous supply of blood, it seems to me that we should be going in a very different direction: trying to reduce the number of people who provide blood, not increase the number. From that perspective, again, we would be paying people for blood and paying more for blood the second and third times that they give, when we are more secure that their blood is safe and healthy.

With regard to finding ways to solve the problem of monitoring blood, much of the problem would have been corrected by making blood suppliers strictly liable for any problems with their blood. Then the incentive is on the blood supplier to monitor and sort in whatever manner they think is appropriate.

I will conclude by saying that these last notions with regard to monitoring are all very interesting. They all suggest different ways in which you would use different kinds of incentives and sorting devices under certain circumstances. An example might be getting donors or vendors through their employers. People who work are generally healthier, more reliable sorts than derelicts. There are many incentives that you can use in which you make use of the market.

My understanding, though, is that all of these concerns now with regard to monitoring are past, that this is something of a dead issue now. My understanding is that over the last 20 years, our ability to lab test the blood has moved to a level where the blood that we actually use is quite safe, regardless of its source. If I am wrong with regard to that, then the monitoring issues come up again. I believe, though, that the safety of our current blood supply is not a function of all of these intrusive prescreening questionnaires that people have come up with, but rather a function of the fact that we can now effectively test for the various forms of hepatitis and HIV. With regard to the letter from the old man that Dr. Westphal read us, that is the reaction you will get from somebody who is donating, who is making a gift. It is not likely to be the reaction you will get from somebody who is trying to sell you something. That is another argument in favor of a market.

QUESTIONS/COMMENTS

Jane Piliavin: I like the way you separate out the selection problem from the lying problem. That is something that is very difficult to do with the kind of correlational data that we have. I do want to point out that consistently to this day, plasma apheresis donors, who are routinely paid, have three times the risk of infectious diseases, as compared to people who are giving their blood. We don't know whether that is selection, lying, or some combination of the two.

Jeffrey McCullough: I would agree with Mr. Cohen about the similarity in the costs of volunteer donors and paid donors, but for a different reason. I think the direct cost to our operation for a paid donor system would be no greater and maybe less than that for the volunteer system because it is a lot easier to call somebody up and get them for pay, so you don't have to shift the cost to the rest of society.

David Jenkins: Red Cross data show that it only costs us about $10 in direct cost to the blood supplier to recruit the donor. That is not taking into account the cost to the companies, which I think is a very important concern. We would have to increase that substantially.

Blood Donor Attitudes and Behavior

Alvin Drake

My involvement with blood donation attitudes and behavior began about 25 years ago, when the Titmuss[4] book, *The Gift Relationship*, appeared. As you may know, it was a book with limited circulation but enormous impact in this country. A rather critical look was taken at our blood collection procedures compared with practices in Great Britain. It described our donors as people, many of whom donated blood for money, and most of whom exhibited a less noble attitude toward social welfare than was the case in Great Britain. As best as I can tell, Titmuss assessed the blood supply in Great Britain by talking to few people and probing not at all deeply into actual donor and blood allocation practices there. The blood supply in the United States was in part assessed by misusing data that I supplied. That certainly got me concerned, curious, and involved.

My earlier work on the blood supply was with technical issues in inventory control, decision making with regard to frozen blood, data handling, and regional sharing. About 20 years ago, we had the days of the American Blood Commission (ABC). People were comparing individual responsibility versus community responsibility. They were really talking about the American Association of Blood Banks versus the Red Cross and were just beginning to recognize blood supply problems that could not be blamed on the public. I was among the early people to contend that much was right with the American blood supply. My claim was that any of us, as patients, should worry a lot more about getting clobbered by triage at an emergency room than about encountering a significant problem meeting our needs for blood. The ABC Donor Recruitment Task Force wondered, among other things, about how much cash and "insurance" incentives compromise the quality of the supply. We could establish that a lot of active, desirable donors said they were much less likely to give blood if they or most other donors were paid.

Ten years ago, we were looking more at significant issues in blood testing and utilization. My research had made me claim that difficulties in places like

---

[4] Titmuss, R (1971). *The Gift Relationship*. New York: Pantheon.

New York City should not be attributed to the contention that New York residents are chronically different from people in Delaware or Minneapolis or Oklahoma. Blood supply problems can result from union contracts and poor recruitment practices, sometimes making collection so expensive that it can't possibly succeed. Today it is nice to hear people emphasize management issues, realizing the blood supply system can be controlled and can perform astoundingly well.

Along the way, some friends and I did a book called *The American Blood Supply*.[5] I would like to tell you a little about that research and its conclusions. With ample funding from NIH, we set out to learn how people feel about the blood supply and to understand the bases of their impressions and decisions about participation or nonparticipation. We picked Hartford, Houston, and New York as cities with very different kinds of blood supplies, from total community responsibility in Hartford to all kinds of things in the other cities. We went after carefully controlled sample populations (using interviewers skilled in seven languages) to learn what we could. We also studied work environments that made it astoundingly easy and routine to be a blood donor, places where you couldn't avoid thinking about blood donation. For this, we went to the big insurance companies in Connecticut, where the odds were that somebody known to an employee would call four times a year to solicit a blood donation. To be a nondonor there, a person would have to have thought out his or her rationale for not donating. That is different from the situation for most nondonors.

We also looked at what happens to high school students at their first opportunity to donate. In addition, we studied samples of very frequent donors, committed nondonors, and ex-donors, to see how they explained their behavior and what may have happened to change it. Our conclusion was (and is) that it is awfully hard to blame the major problems of the blood supply on the general public. We can manage collections better each year to smooth out the supply. But the popular notion that there is a huge crowd of eligible but determined nondonors out there just doesn't hold.

Let me say just a few things about the blood collection task. What is required to meet the needs for whole-blood products, short of what goes into the commercial plasma market? We need every eligible donor in today's population about once every seven or eight years. Of the large population of eligible donors, collections are naturally focused on those who are easily reached and economically drawn.

If too many people were to give their blood, we wouldn't know what to do with it. The number of donors and donations is limited primarily by the

---

[5] Drake, A, S Finkelstein, and H Sapolsky (1982). *The American Blood Supply*. Cambridge, MA: MIT Press.

actual need for blood for transfusion. The issue is how to organize and make collections efficient and predictable, not how to significantly increase the donor base. There may be a larger percentage of active donors in some other countries, but some of their blood can be used for other purposes, maybe providing part of the plasma supply or being drawn for other markets. I doubt that the people in those countries are more or less nice than Americans, though in some cases their collectors may be more organized and/or more subsidized.

In the United States, each year about 10 percent of the people who are eligible to give blood do so. Our donors give an average of about 1.5 donations in a year. That turns out to be around 3.5 percent or so of the total population, including both eligible and ineligible people. It makes no sense to ask why so few people give blood in any one year. We get about what we need. The issue is the hassle, interruption, and economic inefficiencies of the various ways we get the blood we need. What fraction of the people presently eligible to give blood in the United States have ever given blood? Somewhat better than 50 percent. Over a four-year period, probably 25 percent of the eligibles have given at least once. How do people respond to their blood donation opportunities? They respond generously if they are solicited and drawn with respect and convenience. Many will be baffled if you ask them why they donate, so obvious is the need. If you ask donors to select their reasons for blood donation (other than the obvious fact that there are patients who need blood), they will respond with whatever their collector tells them—credits, basic humanity, etc. How do people become ex-donors? Either because of a bad donation experience (long wait, inattention to their treatment, etc.—all fairly rare) or, more usually, either the person moved or the recruitment organization stopped reaching them.

Asking for blood donation reasons can achieve strange results. There was a person at a blood bank who gave blood frenetically, four times a year, maybe five when the number of weeks worked out right. We asked why he did that. He said he gave it for his insurance plan. We replied that he had given eight times as much as required in his blood assurance program. His answer was that people need blood all the time. What did we expect him to do, donate less than he could? Most people don't enjoy blood donation but they are very happy to have participated. We should be careful not to provide potential donors with motivations less solid than those they already have.

How do we convince people to give blood? It is good to sustain an intelligent, continued general awareness of the need. Other factors are invisibly at work favoring the blood supply. For example, by the time a person is 25 years old, the odds are already 50–50 that he or she knows that a personal acquaintance has received a blood transfusion. At age 35, there are three chances out of four that a person is aware of a friend, relative, or other personal acquaintance who has received blood. Collectors sometimes undermine the natural awareness of the need with well-intentioned but personal acquaintance who has received blood. Collectors sometimes undermine the natural awareness of the need with well-intentioned but misleading and sometimes ineffective ads. I'd like to mention one example. There was a big promotion in Massachusetts done by a well-meaning public relations firm that asked too few questions first. Incidentally, it was successful because anything that reminds people to give blood will probably help in the short term, though I believe the long-term costs of misinformation are considerable. The ad went something like this, at least in my unforgiving caricature. "Thump, thump, thump." Heart beating. "Blood is vital for life." Lots of drama and you hear all kinds of noises in the background. "You lose too much of this stuff and you could die. Thump, thump, thump. Nobody will give blood. Thump, thump, thump. So, why don't you?" It is easy to think of more positive messages.

A lot of the ads emphasize that there is a tiny segment of the population—something like 3.5 percent—that gives blood, so why don't you be as heroic as they. There was one campaign with a picture of President Jimmy Carter lying on a table giving his 58th unit of blood. On newsprint, it looked like he was dying. This was part of one of the few national public service Ad Council campaigns. Big stuff. The material gets to be seen and heard by millions of people. But in some of these, there may be 11 sentences in the ad and 10 of them are dead wrong. They would scare me out of giving blood also. People are generous with their blood. People feel good about giving their blood. Treated well and solicited regularly, they will return to give again. If you want to feel good about people, study their attitudes and behavior with regard to blood donation. You'll find them astounding, uplifting and neat.

QUESTIONS/COMMENTS

Lloyd Cohen: The economist reaction generally to the notion that you ask people what they would do under certain circumstances and you take that as a guide is just not a proper way to discover what they are actually going to do. People say all sorts of things. The way to find out what they are going to do is to give them choices. As for the observation that you ask people if they would give blood if they were paid and they say "No," I would have to see it before I would believe it. If it were true, though, my suggestion would be, don't pay those people. Pay other people.

Alvin Drake: I agree that the test is obviously needed. In many cities over long periods of time you did have the choice. The value of the gift to the individual will be significantly undermined if they know that you can go and buy this stuff elsewhere, but I agree that the test isn't being run now. It was run in many places for many years in this country, with some very bad results.

Harvey Klein: I think what you are saying to us is to determine whether or not this is a management problem.

Alvin Drake: I think some excellent things were said earlier about the level to which we delegate recruitment and retention and the way we treat those professionals. I believe it is a management problem. I don't think it is a huge management problem, because if you go around looking for surgeons who say they would have done this and that but they didn't have the blood, you are going to have trouble finding them. We deliver what is needed. Nevertheless, I think that the recruitment and retention function is pushed way down the system where relatively unempowered people try to talk to powerful organizations and get in trouble.

Arthur Bracey: You talked a lot about recruitment. What about the role of public education? Are we trying to educate the public too late? Should we start earlier in school?

Alvin Drake: We have a lot of information on that, but I believe that the most crucial thing for the future of the blood supply is to go after those high schools and colleges tenaciously with people trained to concentrate on those populations. There are problems there. You can get less staff continuity in drive organization. Students are interested in all kinds of things. I saw our blood drive at MIT, which was about the national leader or close to it in per capita units, become just another blood drive when the Red Cross chapter around it collapsed, the chapter having sustained, fed, and paid attention to the students who organized the drive as well as to the donors. I think any system is going to require getting a bunch of blood from young, healthy people and giving it to mostly older people who need blood.

One other thing, though. The general notion that blood donation is important, that you are likely going to need it someday, and that we all have it is good to stress to young adults. We need to tell them that they will feel good for doing it, even though it is somewhat creepy the first time. I think the younger the better. A high school campaign pays off long-term dividends beyond belief. What I remember is that a quarter of the kids eligible in a high school will give at their very first chance. That is amazing. You get in the habit, and I like best that you get in the habit of giving and receiving nothing in return.

III
ENHANCING DISTRIBUTION

American Red Cross Blood Distribution System

Jeany Mark

I would like to talk to you today about the American Red Cross as a total system. We have recently created a "Hub" to increase the availability of blood products by coordinating supply and demand through a consolidated inventory management. One of the things I have been doing this past year is to take a good system, and I believe it is a good system, remove some of the inefficiencies, and then create greater efficiency in what remains. Before I describe that, however, I would like to go over some of our very basic trends to give you a sense of our supply and demand situation with the Red Cross.

We have looked at the average monthly distribution of blood and blood products from 1986 through 1995. The whole blood collections include everything: autologous, allogeneic, and directed. We have taken an average for the past five years and have found that our collections and distributions have matched. The real question here is whether demand drives our collection behavior or whether if we had collected more units of blood, we could have sold them.

The other point that is of interest to our organization is the issue of platelet distribution. Let me just very briefly explain this. From our perspective, we are seeing a substitution effect. That is, as single-donor platelets use increases, random donor platelets usage declines. Interestingly, we used to be growing quite well in apheresis platelets, but it has really been leveling off for our system. If you look at the trend, the total platelet utilization is now tipping downward a little bit.

Moving back to improving the availability of blood, we believe that in our system it is driven mainly by the market demand, blood typing needs, and the dating issue.

The Red Cross whole blood collection has been going down. At one point we used to collect 6.1 million units. Today we are collecting 5.7 million units. However, I believe a lot of the downward trend is driven by autologous and directed donations. Allogeneic collections have been decreasing at a rate of 1/10 of 1 percent on a compound annual growth rate basis, whereas autologous and directed collections have been going down by about 1 percent.

As far as what can we do to increase the availability from a systems perspective, we are looking at coordinating the supply and demand through more of an inventory consolidation, that is, using the Hub concept. The purpose of the St. Louis Hub is to ensure the balance of supply and demand within the ARC as a whole, and to be a single coordinating point for transactions with non-Red Cross blood centers and hospitals. We have restock programs whereby importing ARC centers automatically receive blood products when their inventory levels reach a predetermined threshold. This also obviates the old practice of having to receive unneeded A-positive units in order to get needed O-positive units. Now people can call the Hub and get O's and B's without having to be penalized by having to include and pay for units of other blood that they don't need.

The Hub also plays a role in lessening the impact of unanticipated sharp fluctuations, using some of the odd lots of smaller-unit-volume shipments that you would normally not be able to ship to a big importer such as Los Angeles without incurring a lot of transportation costs. We aggregate them all in the Hub. We have this information in a computer system, and the regions report their inventory level every day.

The other issue that we have is trying to get all of our organizations to adopt uniform definitions of working inventory and critical inventory levels, so that supply can be centrally managed in a much better way than has been done in the past. Today there is still inconsistency in the definitions of these parameters. We now believe the optimal level is three days' worth of inventory. The emergency level is one day's worth. We have been hovering in between the two, that is, between optimal and emergency. There are days that it gets pretty close. I know how it feels when you have 10 units of O-positive on your shelf and you are taking care of 70 hospitals. I know a lot of our blood centers do start to panic then and they do call. But generally when it comes time to really help out, our regions do cooperate and help other regions in dire emergencies.

I mentioned dating as one of the other areas that can increase blood availability. First of all, the restock program provides a much better shelf life. Instead of giving people 15 days to work with, we try to give them a minimum of 36 days. Part of the reason also is that we don't want to have to keep worrying about moving the inventory back and forth, having them order multiple times each week. They also function as a clearinghouse for short-dated products, that is, those units whose shelf life is near expiration. For instance, we get calls from some of our locations in Miami and San Juan requesting blood. We tell them we have some short-dated blood and they take it. We also know certain blood types are less in demand. The one thing that the Hub is trying to do is that instead of moving unneeded short-dated type A units all over the place, we will ship them all in and let them outdate at one place. From a Red Cross perspective, whether it is outdating in Philadelphia or outdating in St. Louis, it doesn't matter to the organization. It is the same dollar amount. Overall, however, the Red Cross system outdates rate has gone down. I don't think that it is due to any particular reason. There are probably a number of reasons over time.

As I mentioned earlier, we currently move blood all over the place, moving most of the red cells from exporting regions to the Hub and then redistributing them to the importing regions. It makes better sense, though, to do direct shipments as much as we can, basically from the exporters to importers. It just doesn't make sense for Philadelphia's imports to come from as far away as Boise, Idaho, when there is a Johnstown Blood Center in Pennsylvania that has the same volume available. We are therefore changing to a "virtual inventory" management system in which the bulk of the products bypass the Hub, which only coordinates and directs the movements.

The other drawback of moving everything through the Hub is that we create an extra day of float that we don't need to do. The newer direct routing takes care of that, and we ultimately save some money, too, by eliminating double shipping.

Our regions have now been regrouped into five areas: Western, South Central, Southeast, North Atlantic, and North Central. The idea is to get each of the areas to be as self-sufficient as possible because they do have a mix of importers and exporters, and where they are short, then we will go through the Hub. Although the Hub will be carrying far less physical inventory, we still want to carry some for emergency purposes, for instance, like the strike that we recently had in one of our locations.

Another area I want to touch upon a little bit is the pricing issue. A year ago, if you looked at the intra-Red Cross movements, prices were all over the place. I would like some of our non-Red Cross friends out there to know that we sell blood cheaper to you than we do to our own partners within the Red Cross system. What we are doing now is standardizing the price. A unit of red blood cells will now be worth the same amount no matter what Red Cross center you buy it from or sell it to. There is no such thing as a markup, so that people won't waste time trying to make the best deal possible. We are focusing on matching supply rather than what is the best deal. As a result, we are in the process of eliminating all the internal billing, where it makes sense, and just do adjustments.

Finally, there are many other future challenges for the Red Cross in its inventory management. One is that we need to have a much better system to manage and forecast the supply and demand.

A second challenge is to better educate the local community about blood not necessarily being a strictly local resource. They may not be willing to help out other blood centers if we cannot overcome the notion that what's collected in their community is strictly for use in their community.

The third challenge is something that the Red Cross will be spending the next 18 months very aggressively working on is driving down some of our costs. I know that there is this issue of whether blood should be treated as a commodity, but I talk to hospital administrators and they tell me they don't care what we have to say, dollars and cents do matter.

QUESTIONS/COMMENTS

Paul Russell: Ms. Mark, you are saying that there needs to be some kind of central coordination within the Red Cross to permit efficient transfer of blood from one distant place to another, and that is not necessarily through your Hub.

Jeany Mark: That is correct. Right now we have a system where everything is actually shipped into St. Louis. We no longer really need to do that. When we have a standardized computer system, it will have a requirement that you can look up each region's inventory level. So, the concept is not to move it physically, but to go point to point.

Paul Russell: Logically speaking, if your approach is as you have described it, then you should also have some kind of oversight about non-Red Cross sources. Are you planning that?

Jeany Mark: Yes. We are talking with the few non-Red Cross partners we have and looking at supplying them. When we need to, we buy from them also.

Paul Russell: Your concept ideally then is of a national system centrally coordinated to include everybody.

Jeany Mark: Yes, that is correct. A week ago we sent out an internal communication to our Red Cross units directing them to refer all blood product transactions with non-ARC centers to the Hub.

Alvin Drake: If hypothetically, then, Dr. Gilcher can supply Los Angeles far less expensively than any Red Cross center, may that happen today or does it have to go through the Hub?

Jeany Mark: Through the Hub. We are trying to manage our own resources so that when there is a demand from outside the Red Cross system, then the Hub makes the call. For example, the Hub calls United Blood Services,

Oklahoma Blood Institute, or other non-ARC blood centers. Likewise, if the non-ARC centers have excess that they want to declare to the Red Cross system, the Hub is the central point for these non-ARC centers to contact. This is the thinking for now, but I see other possible alternatives that may be more effective and strategic to the Red Cross in meeting our customers' demands.

Blood Resource Sharing Programs

Toby Simon

I was very intrigued by the hub concept when the Red Cross put it together. It is interesting that they are now beginning to partially move away from it and toward direct transportation; at United Blood Services (UBS) we couldn't see the economic sense in the double transportation in this age of computers.

We do have a central computer system for United Blood Services, so that we control inventory from a single coordinating position in Scottsdale, Arizona, but we don't physically move the blood into Scottsdale. We move it from its area of availability to its area of need. Like the Red Cross, we have two systems of moving the blood. One is by prearranged agreement. In each budget cycle, those centers that anticipate need provide an estimate of what they will need to import. Those centers that anticipate surplus indicate that, and we try to match it up and have regular commitments through the year.

In addition, we also have on a daily basis the movement of blood from area of oversupply to area of need. That is done by a computer system on which the inventories are pulled up each morning, and the central inventory control person makes certain changes in the morning based the computer display of who has surpluses and who has deficits. Then as the day goes on, he coordinates spot needs that occur. It is on a spot basis that we provide blood outside the system, since we have a surplus and centers, Red Cross or non-Red Cross, elsewhere in the country have needs. We no longer have any special commitments.

We believe that it is ethically and morally appropriate for blood to be shared as a national resource and to go from areas that can draw it more readily to those that have greater needs, whether it is because of a greater concentration of tertiary care centers or other factors. We do believe, however, that a center should never short its own community. So, we have made a special point in the last several years of assuring that any center independently can say, "No, we cannot ship. We cannot meet that commitment because of shortages in our own community." However, there is a strong feeling of camaraderie among our centers, so, just as was mentioned with the Red Cross, people will make that effort, and so generally we meet those needs.

We understand that there is something similar among the Blood Centers of America, a group of independent blood centers that are coordinated in a somewhat looser fashion out of Rhode Island. They have a single system and make both prearranged contractual arrangements through the year and spot arrangements to share blood among participating blood centers.

The major national program is that of the American Association of Blood Banks (AABB), which runs a national blood exchange through its headquarters in Bethesda, Maryland. We participate in that program, which is actually highly efficient and works quite well. We utilize it very extensively, both when we have needs that somehow we can't fill and also when we have surpluses that we want to share with the rest of the country.

There is a little controversy with this system, however, because the AABB will ship a unit, for example, from United Blood Services to a hospital in Boston that is presumably supplied by the American Red Cross or a hospital in New York that is presumably supplied by New York Blood Center. That is somewhat controversial for antitrust reasons and for reasons of the diversity of the AABB membership. The AABB believes that it is obligated to do so on the basis of the fact that these hospitals are members and have qualified for the National Blood Exchange. The antitrust implications stem from the possibility of anticompetitiveness charges if member hospitals are prevented from utilizing this system in lieu of their local blood center. We can talk about that a little more in detail later, but the National Blood Exchange has received a major commitment from the AABB to make blood available as a national resource throughout the country, and many people believe it is highly efficient and highly effective in moving blood from oversupply to undersupply.

The Council of Community Blood Centers (CCCB), of which I am currently president, also runs a program, but it is basically a simple faxnet type of program, whereby if somebody needs blood, it goes over the faxnet and another CCBC member can reply and make the provisions.

In both the AABB and the CCBC, the cost of blood from one center to the other is largely determined by the costs that prevail in the supplying center, and there is a small transactional cost with the National Blood Exchange in order to keep the system afloat. The National Blood Exchange is a managed system with professional management, and the CCBC system right now is not.

American blood policy, which was promulgated in the early 1970s, had two major points, which we have continued to discuss even today at this meeting: regionalization, the concept that there should be a bringing together of hospital needs and supply on a regional basis, and voluntarism. The rational sharing of the national blood resource in a way is an extension of the regionalized concept.

If we do have a national blood resource, where does the blood come from?

I think what we are beginning to see is a coming together of all of the things that we are discussing today because, obviously, you cannot have a sharing if you don't have a collection and an adequate recruitment program. We know that it comes to some extent from rural areas, and I presume that there may be several reasons for this. One is that rural areas have fewer tertiary care centers, so they do not have the transplants or the trauma and may not be offering neonatal intensive care and other kinds of medical care that require large amounts of blood.

They also may have a greater sense of community. We used to have our most successful blood drive in New Mexico in the community of Los Alamos, which is where the atomic bomb was developed. It is 60 miles north of Santa Fe, on a mountain. Once I was telling one of our friends who had lived there what a wonderful thing it is that the community does. "Well," she said, "of course, it is the most exciting thing that happens there all year."

Our most successful recruitment programs are in the Dakotas and Minnesota, very much like the Red Cross. If you look at our Fargo, North Dakota, program, it is highly effective, highly cost-efficient, and the source of a predictable blood supply throughout the year. They use very little fixed-site draw and therefore have lower levels of donor retention than one would expect in this area of the country. Their draw is very heavily based on bloodmobiles in rural areas, which you would think would be costly because you are sending teams out and they stay in hotels. Because that blood supply is so reliable, they actually have an extremely low cost of collection and a very effective program.

On the other hand, our Phoenix blood center has been setting records emphasizing donor retention and fixed sites and reducing their mobile blood drives. Different things work in different areas. We know that rural areas in North Dakota do better than rural areas in Mississippi, Louisiana, and Texas. We assume that some of this has to do with higher educational standards, lower unemployment, and so forth.

Ethnic homogeneity and acculturation are issues that also enter into the equation, and that can be a little bit difficult to discuss, but many of the areas that have been pinpointed as areas of ready supply tend to be more ethnically homogeneous. Perhaps this is related to people's feelings about contributions to the community or sense of community.

One of the interesting points that we can make from United Blood Services concerns our program in New Mexico. The state has the highest ethnic minority population in the country—50 percent Hispanic American and Native American population. While not the highest contributor in the United Blood Services, the program in New Mexico does produce a surplus and shares with other areas of the country. When I discussed the New Mexico donors with our recruiters in the Rio Grande Valley, I told them that obviously one can be successful with Hispanic donors. The recruiters, however, point to the acculturation issue and note that many of their Hispanic donors are new residents of the United States. They haven't built up a sense of community and belonging to the American culture, whereas a large proportion of the Hispanic people in New Mexico have been there for many generations.

Are there also differences between people in different cities in the United States? We have a lot of blood moving into New York, Chicago, and Los Angeles. On the other hand, Houston takes care of its own needs. This year, I sent out certificates to the five UBS centers that set records in 1994. Three of them were where you would expect: Fargo, North Dakota; Rapid City, South Dakota; and Cheyenne, Wyoming. However, two of them were Las Vegas, Nevada, and Phoenix, Arizona, both of which have had a big influx of new residents. So, there are a lot of different factors reacting.

In general, though, we are sending blood to urban areas, where presumably we have a concentration of large tertiary care centers that are heavy utilizers of blood. Where these are not regionalized, we have major problems. If you serve Albuquerque you also serve the whole of New Mexico, which is the referral area for the tertiary care centers. In Albuquerque you would anticipate having an adequate supply, but our friends in Memphis, Tennessee, have blood drives in only a small percentage of the referral area of the hospitals in Memphis. The same is true in Chicago, where both United Blood Services and Life Source are largely limited to the Chicago metropolitan area, although patient referrals may come from southeastern Wisconsin, central Illinois, and so forth.

Ethnic diversity appears to create need and may create blood group-specific problems because the population in need may be of a different group than the donating population. If you are having the people in the Dakotas help people, for example, in Chicago, you will discover that the donors in the Dakotas have a different group distribution than the recipients in Chicago. So, that creates problems in matching supply to utilization.

Now, if we wanted to create a rational distribution, we would presumably move the blood from areas of surplus and areas with lower viral marker rates. We still have a blood center that has yet to have an HIV-confirmed donor, and in general, in areas in the Dakotas and Wyoming or Montana, you have lower marker rates than you have in metropolitan areas such as Miami or Los Angeles. It would seem sensible to make the blood supply safer, move it from areas of lower viral marker rates to areas of higher rates.

Another issue is cost. If we are creating an economically rational distribution system, we are going to have to apply those same techniques on the collection end. That creates an issue because, of course, in moving blood to areas of collection shortfalls and higher viral marker rates, we are most often moving it to higher-cost areas.

Just to give you a little idea of how cost figures into the equation, I asked our chief financial officer to provide me with 1994 data on the cost of producing a unit of red cells in United Blood Services. It goes from less than $50 a unit in North Dakota to more than $80 a unit in California, at least with a lot of factors held constant, such as health insurance for the employees, pension costs, costs of a blood bag, and costs of typing and testing reagents. That difference reflects the costs of operating within different parts of the country and the cost of recruitment: how hard it is to get those donors to come in.

In southern California, where we are required to use nurses and where we have a lot of other requirements, operations are 60 percent more expensive than those in North Dakota. In this day of cost-containment in the hospitals, we are going to be under increasing pressure to move blood from low-cost areas to high-cost areas. What are the implications for our volunteer system? If blood starts to be a commodity and is used for competitive advantage, can we continue to convince volunteer donors to give of themselves and provide blood? All the resource sharing and the distribution problems create ethical concerns on the collection side of the equation.

What we need for distribution is a fully cooperative national system in which we all work together to achieve the safest and most efficient blood supply for the country. If we could move in that direction, we would achieve a great deal for both our donors and our patients. But we do have some hurdles to get over in the current environment. We are under tremendous pressure to produce blood for a lower cost to our hospitals. There will be pressures to move blood from lower-cost areas into higher-cost areas, as well as perhaps more medically defensible requirements or pressures to move blood from lower viral marker areas in rural areas and also to begin to match up the rural areas with the tertiary care areas as well. I think we have a start in this with several national plans, but it would be highly desirable to bring them all together and have full-scale cooperation.

QUESTIONS/COMMENTS

Paul Russell: I gather that there is some connection peripherally between these big systems, one of which you represent, but that, at least to date, there is no central coordination of distribution between systems. You are saying that you would be willing to contemplate that?

Toby Simon: There is some of this through the National Blood Exchange run by the AABB. We have a start of a system, albeit one with some antitrust issues, competition issues, and cost issues. We do have relationships with the Red Cross, although, to be very honest, their Hub concept has impaired those relationships. For example, we wanted to send blood from Ventura County,

California, directly to Los Angeles in order to tell our donors in Ventura County that we are helping Los Angeles, which is where they go for their tertiary care when they need it. The Red Cross, however, wanted the blood sent to the Hub, which removes that connection for our donors and makes it more difficult for us to cooperate. I am delighted to hear that the Red Cross is thinking of changing the nature of the Hub in some areas. We may be able to cooperate more openly and fully.

Exporting Blood from a Regional Blood Center

Ronald Gilcher

So far this afternoon we have heard the approach of the American Red Cross and we have heard Toby Simon talk about United Blood Services, both of which are really multiple blood center systems. In the next few moments I would like to give you the viewpoint of a single exporting regional blood center, the Oklahoma Blood Institute (OBI). We are a single blood center system, but really comprise a total of five blood centers, one very large center in Oklahoma City and four smaller centers, each about a hundred miles away, that do everything that we do the main center except laboratory processing. It is perhaps worth noting that of the 168 people who were killed in that terrible tragedy that we recently suffered in Oklahoma City, there were 149 adults, and of those 149 adults, 50 were donors in our system. So, essentially 33 percent of those people were active donors in our system. I think that is an astounding number.

The Oklahoma Blood Institute started in 1977, and I came on board as its director two years later. It was clear to me when I arrived in Oklahoma City that this center was not going to survive unless it could achieve self-sufficiency. Between 1977 and 1981, the Oklahoma Blood Institute imported as much as 40 percent of its blood supply. It was obvious that we had to reverse that, and we finally achieved what we called self-sufficiency by August of 1981. That was the last time that our system had to make an appeal for blood through the media. Indeed, by 1983, using the same principles that we used to achieve self-sufficiency, we became an exporting center or a resource-sharing center able to draw about 30 percent more blood than what we need for use within our system.

There are three critical issues in health care and also in transfusion medicine. The major focus in this country today is on the *cost* of the system. The other two are *availability* (supply or access to medical care) and *quality*, with its associated safety and regulatory issues. I want to keep each of those in perspective during the remainder of this talk.

As we achieved self-sufficiency at the Oklahoma Blood Institute, we determined our requirements for each blood product. Our system is somewhat unique in that all of the platelets and all of the plasma that are now used within our system come from a relatively small group of pedigreed donors. We have approximately 5,000 donors who are supplying over 30,000 products in terms of plasma and platelets. That puts us in a position to be able to export platelets from whole blood and then plasma from whole blood either as fresh frozen or as recovered. So, all of the platelets and all of the plasma in our system are now from single-donor sources.

What we have done is to add 10 percent to what we believe we would need to supply our area. This covers incompletes, laboratory losses, and outdates. Interestingly, our outdates are extremely low, with red cells running about 0.5 to 0.7 percent. Then we added an additional 20 percent as a buffer—for emergencies or other sudden high use. What is critical to us as a single system is that if we don't use that much, we have to market it outside of our area or our costs would be driven up. These blood products become available for ad hoc out-of-region use if they are not used within our region. Our needs of course will vary during the year. For example, our biggest problem in terms of reducing our supply is what we call natural events. If we get ice or snow in Oklahoma City, that knocks our draw way down, but virtually nothing else really reduces our draw.

As we were in the process of increasing our collections, we were able to continue to turn on our donor base and get additional collections for out-of-region use. Basically, most of this was on a contract basis with other regional blood centers or in some cases hospitals. Our purpose was to do this with other regional blood centers. Essentially we became an overcollector and our overcollection amounts to almost 30,000 units of blood per year. When you add ad hoc sales onto that, it would bring us at times essentially to having 40,000 units of red cells available over the course of a year.

If you meet the three issues of cost, supply, and quality as a regional blood center, there really is very little, if any, reason for a hospital within your system to look or go elsewhere. That means you must maintain communications with those hospitals. Just last week a large hospital in New York City called us and wanted us to become a direct supplier. I said we don't want to do that. We would much rather deal with the regional blood center. I asked why they were not talking with the New York Blood Center, and they said they had but they weren't listened to. And as a result of breakdown in communications, they were now looking elsewhere.

There is also what I call value added, and that is where the blood center, for example, manages the inventory. We do that within our system. There is no outdate at our hospitals. No hospital in our system outdates a unit. If it happens, it is our fault, not theirs.

Medical consultation is readily available. We adhere to this by having a small number of physicians who are on call essentially 24 hours a day and we do stick to that. We are readily available within our system.

The blood center also handles all of the other special needs, such as red cell, white cell, platelet, and reference issues. We try to make it a lot easier for the hospitals. Ultimately, what we would like to do within our system is move toward the concept of the centralized transfusion service. It is clearly the way for us to move in the future.

What are some of the pros and cons of overcollection? It is very clear that the economies of scale play a role here. We are clearly in a position of overcollecting red cells, and that has allowed us to do things that we could not have done if we were a smaller organization, in terms of the quality of our staff, our laboratories, and certainly some of the research that goes on in-house.

Clearly, it has made us more cost-effective. The increased revenues have allowed us to do a variety of other things. But there are also areas in the country where this blood is needed, and that puts us in a unique position of being able to share resources. We try to make our donor population aware of the fact that we are resource sharing, and they are very proud of the fact that Oklahomans can help other places in the country. For example, about a week and a half ago, there was a minor catastrophe with a computer system in a large regional blood center in a southern city. On that day they had no platelets that they could pull out of their inventory to send out. They called on us, and we were able to immediately ship in about 15 to 20 units of single-donor platelets out of our inventory because we maintain a minimum of 40 to 100 units of single-donor platelets at all times.

What are the cons of overcollection? One of the cons is that when you make a contract with a regional blood center or a hospital, you have a responsibility to provide. That means that there is pressure on us to draw that extra blood in order to meet that responsibility. What is another con? If you lose the contract, then you have to go out looking for another contract to fill that void or the costs in your system go up because even though you decrease the amount of blood that you draw, you still have overhead requirements.

Another issue is that of locating customers. Actually, we don't locate customers because they come to us. We prefer to work with the regional blood center. The calls come into OBI, and it is the reputation of availability that brings in the calls. Hospitals that are dissatisfied with the regional blood center initiate a call to OBI for ad hoc or contract blood products. We do work with regional blood centers, and we are dealing with some hospitals directly, although we prefer not to. The problem is that the hospitals are constantly calling us because they have some dissatisfaction with the primary blood center. Part of this really inadvertently comes about because of working through the National Blood Exchange.

Because the National Blood Exchange is not only dealing with the regional blood center, but, in fact, even more so with the hospital, one is put into the situation where, because OBI is dealing with the National Blood Exchange, it becomes an OBI-hospital relationship through the National Blood Exchange.

In summary, when the hospitals are dissatisfied with the regional blood center because of price or because of availability—and that is really what it comes down to, those two issues today—they will go to someone outside the system, someone who is known to have blood available. Indeed, that is the way our system has evolved. It has been cost-effective for us to do that. We have become known as a blood center that has an excess of all types of products available, from single donor products to whole blood-derived products.

QUESTIONS/COMMENTS

Robert Travis: Does your no-outdate policy also apply to apheresis products?

Ronald Gilcher: Yes, it does. We require a hospital that has an aging unit of single-donor platelets to send it back to us or let us know when it has two days left on it. We can move the product, some of it, if it has 48 hours left on it.

Paul Russell: Dr. Gilcher, I presume this excess in blood means that your transactions keep you in the black. Right?

Ronald Gilcher: Not necessarily. We would like it to be that way, but there are clearly times that we fluctuate back and forth. We operate with really a very narrow amount of revenue over expense. Interestingly, for the 1994–1995 year we operated slightly in the red.

Paul Russell: I don't say that in criticism. That is a perfectly American thing to do, to operate in the black. I was just curious about how it happens because I think many of the other people operate in a somewhat different fashion.

Henrik Bendixen: I have a related question, which is that the processing taking place in a modern blood center relies on very expensive equipment, including computers and so forth. What is the minimum throughput that you need in order to meet the cost of operating the center?

Ronald Gilcher: That is an extremely important question. That is the whole issue of the economies of scale. I am a great believer in redundancy and backup. I am sure many of you in this room are as well, but if you are a small blood center, the costs of redundancy and backup become incredibly high. We have duplication on everything in our system or even triplication when it comes to our computer system. It is a unique system that was developed in-house. It is a dual mainframe with a third computer that handles distribution, so we are virtually never down.

I would say that one has to exceed 100,000 units per year to be in the situation we are in. Our whole blood throughout between allogeneic, directed, and autologous is about 130,000 units, and our single donor products, platelets and plasma, add about another 30,000. Our total throughput thus approaches 160,000 donations.

We want a system that is steady all year long, and we really are very close to doing that. Even though in-house usage may fluctuate, our draw is very steady for the whole year. We plan to draw extra, for example, during holiday times because we know that there are other places in the country that will want blood products. We wouldn't have to do that, but we plan and plan when it comes to the recruitment area and, in fact, are effective in drawing blood as we have planned.

Jeany Mark: You mentioned that when a hospital's criteria for cost, quality, and availability are met that it will not switch blood suppliers. However, the cost is not fixed. The threshold is constantly getting lowered. I am curious whether you are seeing the phenomenon that I am seeing in some of our centers, one of which recently got back five hospitals that it had previously lost, and in the magnitude of 20,000 units. Do you see that happening?

Ronald Gilcher: My personal belief is that we cannot raise the price on blood products. In fact, this year we reduced our prices. That is part of the reason that we operated in the red for 1994 and 1995. However, we are looking at other sources of revenue that are unrelated to blood products; that is, testing and other areas that I won't go into, that will enhance the revenue stream of the organization. That is critical, as is becoming more cost-effective.

Supply and Demand in Transfusion Services

Arthur Bracey

I come today as a user of blood. In fact, at my facility we transfuse about 50,000 components a year. What I will try to do is to give you the transfusion service perspective on the issues of supply and demand.

We should know, based upon the blood orders that come into the transfusion service, what our inventory needs are. Unfortunately, we aren't in a system where we get blood orders far in advance. In elective surgery, we find out about the surgery schedule sometimes 6 hours, sometimes 12 hours ahead of time. If we could find out further in advance when elective surgery is scheduled, we could have a better-coordinated system for projecting daily blood demands. In addition, we have inventories of blood in our hospitals, which are known largely only to the hospitals and are often unknown to the blood centers. In this day of computerization, one would think that in many centers the hospital inventories could be monitored on a periodic basis with an electronic process that allows data to be fed into the regional blood center for assessment of regional inventory. In fact, such a system could facilitate estimation of the national inventories and resource sharing.

The problem is that the exchange of information is not routine. In my area exchange of inventory data is crisis driven. I find out about a blood shortage when it is there. I don't find out about an impending blood shortage. Part of the problem is also that we are stuck with old techniques. We still exchange data primarily by telephone conversation, not by computers.

In a transfusion service, we often have marked fluctuations in blood needs. For instance, we had a case on Wednesday of a woman who had a placenta previa and suddenly dropped from a hemoglobin of 14 g/dl to a hemoglobin of 5 g/dl. The prospect of such an urgent situation demands that we stockpile blood in order to be sure of meeting all patient needs.

The question that comes up is how efficient are we at determining the stockpile? We have talked today about meeting the inventory needs of transfusion services, but no one has talked about critically assessing how that need is determined. Important factors in determining inventory requirements include the institution's approach to providing blood for patients, that is, the crossmatch-to-transfusion (CT) ratio, the length of time units of blood are held in reserve, and other factors that are management issues from the perspective of a hospital transfusion service.

Unfortunately, by virtue of its perishable nature, blood has a limited life span that affects its availability. There has been work done largely out of the New York Blood Center addressing inventory modeling based upon evaluation of wastage versus shortage of blood products. If we look at my institution's usage on a day-to-day basis (see Table 4), there are peaks and valleys. On the weekends, we need much less blood than we need on routine workdays. Our surgeons like to operate Monday through Wednesday. They take off early on Friday. Saturday and Sunday are low-volume days. Thus, we have data that allow us to anticipate when our peaks and valleys will occur. We look at the efficiency of the use of inventory as a function of outdate, but is that really the correct answer? Is that the correct approach to determining the efficiency of inventory management?

TABLE 4: Red Blood Cell Use (units) at St. Luke's Episcopal Hospital by Day of the Week

Week Number	Mon	Tues	Wed	Thurs	Fri	Sat	Sun
1	101	68	45	55	37	20	42
2	69	68	123	66	37	34	67
3	75	78	69	63	46	24	49
4	88	105	103	54	51	17	27
5	61	65	68	69	42	30	70
6	98	115	88	107	41	32	62
7	59	75	69	74	38	29	52
8	105	60	76	116	47	19	120
Mean	82	79	80	76	42	26	61
Std Dev	17	19	23	22	5	6	26

Inventory is assessed largely by blood wastage and blood shortage data, that is, inability to support a patient need. Ideally, the inventory requirements should be set by historical transfusion volume and case demand. I am not sure, however, how often that happens. A real challenge that we face in transfusion medicine is that of improving our efficiency of inventory management. I know that a person having a cardiac bypass procedure will use 2.2 units. I am trying to learn how much blood a nonsurgical patient with lung cancer will use. We have been most successful at predicting the surgical blood need, but I think we have a lot to learn as far as estimating nonsurgical blood need and nonsurgical case volume. I want to emphasize that many studies assessing surgical blood support have been published, but many facilities are not using them in determining inventory levels.

Sinelson and Bradheim's work on inventory management is interesting.[6] Their model is based upon analysis of the normalized stock level, which is a function of blood stock divided by the mean daily usage. They developed a formula to predict the interaction of outdate and shortage based upon selected normalized stock levels. The formula, in fact, when applied to real hospitals, proved accurate in predicting shortage and outdate. The problem here is that you have to have set points for acceptable frequencies of outdate and shortage. In routine transfusion service practice, many directors have no input regarding these set points and may be unaware of any such determinations by others. From the perspective of a transfusion service, the blood centers which could be helpful are often underinvolved in helping to set transfusion service blood inventory levels.

If the director of a transfusion service wants to be safe and avoid any blood shortages, he can just stockpile enough blood to be sure he will never run out. Of course, as you decrease the amount of the normalized stock ratio, which is the amount of stock related to the mean daily demand, there will be an increasing frequency of shortage.

There is another important consideration. Blood that is out in the field may not be being used appropriately. We feel we have shortages on the regional and national levels, but we often have maldistribution of blood rather than true shortage. The places that have a small mean daily transfusion have a real problem in avoiding excessive blood outdating. Likewise, it is inefficient for a hospital to keep blood crossmatched for three days. Thus, in hospitals it is very important to look at issues of crossmatch-to-transfusion ratio. In the transfusion service, we can't really impact the shelf-life of the blood, but we certainly can manage certain variables, such as how long we will keep blood crossmatched. When you have centralized facilities where transfusion support care of many patients is taking place, you have economies of scale which mitigate against blood maldistribution.

With respect to shortage, there is a convergence in the curves predicting shortage frequency as you keep less blood. If you have a normalized stock ratio of about 1.5, you begin to experience a significant amount of shortage, but, again, what is shortage? Shortage is having to call the blood center to ask it to provide blood. If more blood is available at the blood center and the

---

[6] Sinelson, V and E Bradheim (1991). A computer planning model for blood platelet production and distribution. *Computer Methods and Programs in Biomedicine, 35:* 279–290.

transportation system is efficient, then this situation really isn't a problem since it doesn't impact patient care. However, this scenario demands an efficient transportation system. If I need a unit of blood urgently, I don't want to hear that it is going to come in two hours. I would rather hear it will be delivered in 15 minutes. From the perspective of the transfusion service, I don't want to call various hospitals or regional blood centers when I need support. I want one number to call and I want the blood in 20 minutes. That is all I want.

Prior to the era of Good Manufacturing Practices (GMP) as directed by the FDA, blood was available at an earlier time following collection. In my area, by 8:00 A.M. we could inventory blood that had been drawn on the preceding day. Post-GMP, the blood is available at noon, but what surgery starts at noon? This delay is particularly an issue with units that have a shorter shelf-life, such as platelets.

Will centralized donor testing further decrease the responsiveness of the blood centers to provide that urgent need that we have? If you don't have a good transportation system, there will be unnecessary stockpiling. So, the system needs to be focused on rapid and efficient provision of blood products. What about remote depots? That was tried in our region, and it cost more because someone had to man the post 24 hours a day. I don't know if it could work, except maybe in places such as Alaska, where remote depots may be the only acceptable alternative.

When there is a shortage in a blood transfusion service, you are always wondering in the back of your mind if the first order always gets delivered first. I still don't know that answer. Another question is whether blood orders are related to real need. Are the inventories fairly and equitably distributed? Again, what is most important is speedy and reliable delivery. Blood products have got to be there when you need them.

Return policy is another issue. I understand a blood center discouraging return of short-dated blood, but I just don't understand some return policies. Currently in our region, if you order leukocyte-reduced blood, you can't return it, despite its long shelf life. I don't understand the reason for that policy when you can return other sorts of blood. Some policies impede the free interchange of blood, which is important in facilitating distribution.

There is also the issue of the delivery fee. If you are going to charge large sums to have blood delivered, then people will stockpile the blood, potentially keeping more blood available than they need. Blood products need to be made readily available and transported without exorbitant fees.

There was a study in Sydney, Australia, of a blood center's role and what it could do when it got involved with the hospitals in the region to improve inventory management. The blood outdate rate dropped from 5 percent to 0.9 percent after implementation of an educational effort. Factors that were found to be important in this particular study included: (1) whether or not the hospital had a functioning rather than a perfunctory transfusion committee; (2) smaller hospitals had greater problems with outdates and management of inventories; (3) CT ratio greater than 2 was found to be a significant problem with respect to outdate; and (4) those institutions that were remote kept more blood and outdated more blood.

The Wall Street Journal recently reported that 20 percent of hospitals that transfuse autologous blood have mistakenly given allogeneic blood prior to transfusing the intended autologous blood. These errors occur because we often have these special requests, but no fail-safe way to link the patient and his autologous unit in a definitively positive manner. Some system needs to be developed to positively track these units from collection through infusion.

There is also the issue of giving group-matched platelets to people who routinely request them. Some physicians will only give Type A platelets to Type A individuals and they won't give Type O platelets to Type A individuals. How much are you letting your consumers drive inefficient blood practices? We do have special requests on occasion. For instance, we may need a lot of antigen-negative blood when we are transfusing either multiple alloimmunized patients or patients in whom we are trying to prevent multiple alloimmunization. This is another area where our blood center can help us a great deal by providing appropriate antigen-matched blood.

Finally, I will make one last comment. When I go to the supermarket to buy milk, I consciously look for the milk with the longest shelf life. You wonder what happens in the transfusion services when staff members are ordering blood from the blood center. Is it the individual facility's benefit that is overriding, or is it the public or the greater benefit? I don't know, but my milk analogy makes me wonder.

QUESTIONS/COMMENTS

Robert Travis: Just a curiosity question. Out of any given hundred days, how many days is your inventory at your optimal level?

Arthur Bracey: Good question. I would say that we are at our optimum level about 60 percent of our days.

Logistic Problems and Perishables: The Kroger Company and Supermarket Seafood

Robert Fields

The Kroger Company is the largest grocery retailer in the United States. We have about 1,200 stores spread out over 20 different states all over the country. We buy and ship over one billion pounds of perishable product annually, and that perishable product has a shelf life from 3 days up to about 45 days for cheese and processed products. Thus, we have a tremendous jigsaw puzzle that we are putting together every day.

I am responsible for all the procurement aspects of all the meat commodities and categories in our Kroger stores. I am also responsible for all the quality assurance procedures and also for following up on distribution for getting all the meat all over the country. There are a lot of similarities between what we do at Kroger and what you do with the blood supply. I will give you an example of how we are solving some of the logistic problems, some of the waste problems, and some of the distribution problems we have out there.

In terms of compliance and safety issues, we deal with the USDA, the FDA, local and state agriculture departments, and local health departments. We have a series of procedures and guidelines that we have to follow. One of the problems that we deal with is that different health departments have different guidelines. We are constantly having to work under all the realms. Sometimes we even have instances in which the USDA or federal regulatory committee will have one set of rules, but a state or a local agency will knock those out and impose their own rules. Sometimes there is even some one-upsmanship or some competition. To combat that and to guarantee that we are in compliance with all the regulations and procedures, the Kroger Company has developed one of the most thorough quality assurance programs in the industry. We have quality assurance staffs in each of our marketing areas. We are constantly evaluating product quality coming into our distribution centers. We are also constantly going out to the stores and monitoring quality levels out there, monitoring temperature, shelf life, and all types of bacteria.

We also have a corporate staff in Cincinnati, which talks directly with Washington, D.C., and communicates all the new regulations out to the stores.

I would like to concentrate today on our distribution and merchandising principles for the seafood department that might apply to your business. Much like your blood supply and blood usage, there isn't any demand pattern or supply pattern. Because seafood is an industry that still depends upon a hunted species, we can't count on our supply at any one point in time. Also, we never know what the customers are going to want in our stores. In many regards, then, our selling pattern varies widely, just like your blood supply.

Price fluctuation is another comparison area. I understand that pricing is not level in your industry. Similarly, in seafood our prices can fluctuate 10 to 40 percent in a matter of days. In one or two days, it can go up a dollar or two dollars a pound.

One of the challenges that we are looking at in seafood is the huge swing in supply and demand. Another key issue is temperature control. It is one of the most important areas in controlling quality and safety. We must keep our seafood products under 35°F, and the colder we can keep them, the longer the shelf life and the higher the quality we can maintain. Fresh seafood typically has seven days of shelf life from when it hits the docks. We have to be able to push that product through our entire system and still leave a couple days for the consumer's refrigerator, to ensure the quality level.

Product cost varies. We may have set a retail price for sole in our stores of $6.99 a pound. If the market fluctuates the next day and our cost goes up, we have basically lost all of our margin. Thus, fluctuation is a big problem for us. In addition, we are trying to guess what the customer is going to buy. We have the same inventory problems that you have. We are putting seafood out in the case, not knowing what is going to sell that day. Our seafood shops are operating more or less as a convenience to the consumer.

Our waste in our actual stores can sometimes hit 20 to 25 percent. That was a critical point that we had to address. How do we lower the waste in our stores? Our solution was a new type of distribution network. Distribution for us involves taking products from Canada, Mexico, the Gulf of Mexico, the Northeast, and South America and distributing them over 1,200 grocery stores in 20 states. That is a logistical nightmare. Until recently, what we were doing was a little bit like the Red Cross scenario. We had a hub, which was at our Greensburg Seafood Distribution Plant. We would bring all the products into that distribution facility, spread them out to different regional warehouses, and then once again put them on another truck and put them into the stores. We were cross-trucking product four or five times before it actually got to the store. We have been in discussions with people at Emery Air Freight, and they created a tremendous software and technology package for us. With it we are going to forward contract with our suppliers in different regions. We will negotiate costs, product specs, and supplier or inventory deliveries.

Once those negotiations are completed, Emery is going to tie in with our individual store ordering system via satellite. Each store is going to be able to scan a little bar code or a special number that is going to indicate, say, Dover sole. That order will be transmitted via satellite to Emery, which will basically be our hub, and then Emery will automatically throw that out to the suppliers.

Those suppliers will get the product, Emery will arrange pickup, and that product will be delivered directly to our stores through Emery. The key advantage to this system is that we can order a product at 2 P.M. today and have guaranteed delivery of that product into our stores by 11:30 A.M. the next day. We have reduced four days worth of float on all the products we had going all over the system. That is inventory management. There is a lot of money saved on that, and we have added four days of shelf life to our product where it needs to be, right there in front of the consumer.

In turn, we are going to reduce our waste. We think we are going to reduce our waste by half right off the bat, and hopefully knock it down to somewhere around 5 to 7 percent. Another big advantage is that we are able to give our consumers the variety they need instantly. If a customer comes in and needs a special request, it currently takes four to five days to get it. Now, it will only take 24 hours.

Basically, that is what we are doing in the distribution network, but there are a couple of comments I wanted to make. Our customers are just like your donors in a lot of ways. One of the things that we found out is that to keep a customer will cost a dollar, but to bring a customer back costs you 10 dollars. Just as with your donors, it is very important to keep that customer because in the long run it is going to save money. Another thing that we demand of our stores is that they treat the customer like you would want to be treated yourself. That helps us keep that customer there.

QUESTIONS/COMMENTS

Paul Russell: Do you ever get a product out in one of your stores and notice that it is not selling there, and think it ought to be in Cincinnati or somewhere else?

Robert Fields: Not in the seafood scenario. With beef or some longer-shelf-life items, I might transfer them over to another division. What makes that possible is we have a centralized procurement department that coordinates all that effort out to all the different places. We'll be able to do it even better with our satellite system.

Peter Logue: When you do transfer that product, do you lower the cost to the customer, as it is now, I would assume, not as fresh?

Robert Fields: We are operating all the stores under the same umbrella. It is the Kroger Company, and basically we pass on the same cost that that division bought it at to the next division. There are limits of course. We are not going to send a problem to another division and create another problem. Your first loss is your best loss, so if you are going to have to discount, you might as well do it in the division where the problem began.

William Sherwood: It sounds like your transportation company, Emery, is going to manage the whole inventory for your seafood business to the point of buying and selling and shifting and making all the decisions because they have the computer system.

Robert Fields: They have the technology. That is correct. The Kroger Company is going to continue to negotiate cost and product specifications, but Emery is going to turn into more or less an order placer, which will take the orders from my stores and distribute them out to different suppliers.

IV
EXPANDING THE ALTERNATIVES

Frozen Red Cell Technology

C. Robert Valeri

Although I was invited here today to talk about frozen blood, it is not actually the blood that is frozen, but just specific cells in the blood, so what I will brief you on today is the status of red blood cell (RBC) freezing. The most common approach to the freeze-preservation of red blood cells in the United States today is accomplished primarily using high concentrations (40% weight/volume [w/v]) of intracellular glycerol as a cryoprotectant and storage with mechanical refrigeration at -80°C. Originally, there was a great effort to use low concentrations (20% w/v) of glycerol and freezing at -150°C, which was achieved with liquid nitrogen. I understand that this costly system is now being phased out and that the Europeans, primarily the British Army, are presently interested in using extracellular hydroxyethyl starch as the cryoprotectant because postthaw washing would not be required. Glycerol is the most widely used cryoprotectant, but the previously frozen red blood cells must be washed before transfusion to remove the glycerol. Postthaw washing is the major logistic problem with freezing red blood cells with glycerol, whether you use high or low glycerol; postthaw washing to reduce glycerol to less than 1 gram percent is necessary. Although red blood cells frozen with hydroxyethyl starch do not require washing, this method is not a popular one.

The types of red blood cell products we have been freezing at the Naval Blood Research Laboratory over the past 20 years through the support of the U.S. Navy are as follows:

- Nonrejuvenated: The major frozen red cell inventory, autologous and rare blood.
- Indated-Rejuvenated: Red cells with improved oxygen transport function.
- Outdated-Rejuvenated: Red cells salvaged from outdated blood supply.
- Quarantine: All cryopreserved red blood cells can be used as a source of quarantined allogeneic red blood cells.

We freeze nonrejuvenated red blood cells shortly after blood collection while the oxygen transport function of the red blood cells is still maintained. For obvious reasons, this method is used primarily for the freeze-preservation of autologous red cells and rare red cells. We have also been rejuvenating O-positive and O-negative donor red blood cells prior to freezing to restore or improve their oxygen transport function, which deteriorates during liquid storage. The reason that only O-positive and O-negative red cells are rejuvenated and frozen for allogeneic use is that the problems associated with thawing, washing, and postwash storage, which I will discuss, make the practice not feasible for other than O-positive and O-negative red blood cells.

Our laboratory became interested in the rejuvenation process during the Vietnam War when we recognized that there were large quantities of outdated O-positive and O-negative red blood cells in Vietnam. We developed a procedure for rejuvenating not only outdated red cells but indated red cells as well. Rejuvenation of indated red cells improves the oxygen transport function of the red cell, a very important benefit in specific clinical situations.

Previously frozen red cells are used in at least the following seven ways:

1. Autologous: anticipated surgery.
2. Autologous: potential future use, insurance to minimize use of allogeneic blood.
3. Quarantined allogeneic O-positive and O-negative red cells can be frozen for greater than 6 months, during which time the donor can be retested for infectious disease markers.
4. Rare type and selected red cells can be saved.
5. Red cells with improved oxygen transport function are especially useful in coronary artery and cerebrovascular disease, cardiopulmonary bypass surgery, and hypothermia.
6. Patients with immunoglobin A (IgA) deficiency and paroxysmal nocturnal hemoglobinuria (PNH).
7. Rare and autologous red cells can be refrozen after thawing.

The most important of these uses is the quarantine of allogeneic frozen red cells, i.e., the use of freeze-preservation as a means of avoiding the potential for transmission of disease through an allogeneic transfusion. It is now possible to quarantine frozen donor red blood cells for at least 6 months to retest the donor for pathogens that were undetectable at donation.

As Table 5 shows, however, transfusion of long-frozen red blood cells within 24 hours of thawing is feasible even after storage for up to 21 years.

TABLE 5 Experience with Long-Term Frozen Storage of Red Blood Cells Transfused Within 24 hours of Thawing

Method	Material Preserved	Frozen Storage Limit
-150°C liquid nitrogen, hydroxyethyl starch (HES)	Nonrejuvenated RBCs	Limited data
-150°C liquid nitrogen, 20% (w/v) glycerol	Nonrejuvenated RBCs	At least 8 yrs
-80°C mechanical refrigeration, 40% (w/v) glycerol	(a) nonrejuv RBCs; (b) indated rejuv RBCs; (c) outdated rejuv RBCs	At least 21 yrs; At least 14 yrs; At least 14 yrs
-80°C mechanical refrigeration, 6% DMSO	Platelets	At least 2 yrs
-80°C mechanical	Plasma	At least 7 yrs

The major problem that the military frozen blood banking system faces today is the limited postthaw storage period. At the present time, the FDA approves a postthaw storage period of only 24 hours because of fear of contamination. In our laboratory, we use a sodium chloride-glucose solution during deglycerolization and postthaw storage, and we have data collected over the past 20 years that indicate that washed previously frozen red blood cells can be stored safely at 4°C in a sodium chloride-glucose solution for at least seven days. Moreover, when we used an additive solution such as ADSOL (AS-1), Optisol (AS-5), or Nutricel (AS-3), all currently approved for liquid storage, we observed acceptable 24-hour posttransfusion survival values, acceptable residual hemolysis, and no contamination, even after 2 weeks of postthaw storage at 4°C.

Our primary goal now is to help develop a closed system for the deglycerolization procedure to insure sterility for two weeks at 4°C and gain FDA approval for a longer postthaw storage period. I want to stress again that what I am talking about are allogeneic O-positive and O-negative red blood cells only.

I would like to comment briefly here about the frozen blood banking system deployed by the Department of Defense that uses a -80°C mechanical freezer with an air-cooled dual-cascade compressor requiring 230 volts. We have gained FDA approval for storage of nonrejuvenated red blood cells frozen with 40% w/v glycerol in these freezers for 10 years. Actually, we have studied nonrejuvenated frozen red blood cells after 21 years of frozen storage and have published data showing satisfactory results.

We have also frozen both indated and outdated rejuvenated red cells which have been approved by FDA for storage at -80°C for 10 years. These are red blood cells that are biochemically modified to restore or improve their oxygen transport function before freezing with 40% w/v glycerol. These frozen red blood cells have been stored in -80°C mechanical freezers for at least 14 years with satisfactory results. The U.S. Navy has -80°C mechanical freezers aboard ships as well as at mobile hospitals. These freezers maintain supplies of frozen platelets as well as the frozen O-positive and O-negative allogeneic red blood cells with normal or improved oxygen delivery capacity. Platelets are frozen with dimethylsulfoxide (DMSO), an FDA-approved cryoprotectant. Frozen platelets can be stored at -80°C for at least two years.

We are also able to freeze pluripotential mononuclear cells for use in bone marrow transplantation: these cells can be frozen with 10 percent DMSO and stored at -80°C for 1.5 years. We have also received FDA approval for the storage of fresh frozen plasma at -80°C for seven years.

To summarize the data: the -80°C mechanical freezer can be used by the Department of Defense to store frozen red cells for 21 years, frozen platelets for 2 years, frozen pluripotential mononuclear cells for 1.5 years and fresh frozen plasma for 7 years.

Dr. Fratantoni has asked me to comment on justification for the use of frozen red blood cells, since as we heard earlier from Dr. McCullough, it is quite costly. I have already listed the various uses for frozen red blood cells. I believe the importance of these uses justifies the additional cost for freezing O-positive and O-negative allogeneic red blood cells, selected red blood cells, rare red blood cells, and autologous red blood cells. We have found that patients undergoing specific surgical procedures require red blood cells with the ability to deliver more oxygen to tissue at high oxygen tensions. Before the storage limit of liquid preserved red blood cells was extended to 42 days and before mandated testing of blood products for the infectious disease markers for hepatitis B and C and HIV, there was an interest in freezing autologous red cells. Although the fear of transmission of disease is not as great as it was prior to 1985, freezing O-positive and O-negative donor red blood cells for a 6-month quarantine period would allow time for the donor to be retested to document the presence or absence of infection at the time of retesting.

I would now like to describe to you one of the latest work efforts in our laboratory which I consider to be important. As you have heard, there is a large supply of outdated Type A and Type B red blood cells. We have been investigating a procedure introduced several years ago by Jack Goldstein at the

New York Blood Center to enzymatically convert B and A red blood cells to O red blood cells. Studies are in progress to assess enzymatically converted B and A red blood cells to O red blood cells which are then biochemically modified and frozen with 40% w/v glycerol and stored at -80°C in mechanical freezers.

I'll close by describing probably one of the most important areas of investigation at our laboratory at the present time: the development of closed automated deglycerolization methods. The FDA mandated that a sterile docking device must be used to dock the thawed units to the washing system. The FDA has also recommended that the deglycerolization solutions be passed through 0.22 micron filters, which will require an automated system. To accomplish these goals, the U.S. Army and the U.S. Navy are both working with three commercial companies which have contracts to develop a closed deglycerolization system. The success of this project would allow postwash storage of deglycerolized red blood cells for at least two weeks at 4°C.

QUESTIONS/COMMENTS

Pinya Cohen: What is the cost of initially freezing the red blood cells, then of deglycerolizing them later?

C. Robert Valeri: I would say that the total cost of providing previously frozen red blood cells is three times the cost of liquid preservation.

Pinya Cohen: What I am wondering is the need for extending the frozen storage at -80°C from 10 years to 20 years.

C. Robert Valeri: The extension of frozen storage from 10 years to 20 years would avoid the need to discard the frozen glycerolized red blood cells after 10 years. It means that you have to replace the supply in the freezers, which is costly for the government. If you could store the red cells for 20 years, the costs would be less. In our experience the cost for freezing, thawing, and washing is three times the current cost of collecting and storing red cells in the liquid state.

Pinya Cohen: Do you have a breakdown of cost of thawing and washing independent of the freezing?

C. Robert Valeri: Yes. What we did several years ago, which I really didn't emphasize, was to design a method to freeze the red cells in the same bag in which they were collected With this method, the freezing of the red cells represents a relatively small percentage of the total cost. The major costs associated with freezing are those for the instruments used in processing and the disposables and solutions. So, actually, about 20 percent of the total cost is related to the freezing of the red cells.

Pinya Cohen: So, from that perspective then, the only advantage to expanding it from 10 years to 20 years or whatever has nothing to do with the deglycerolization. It has to do with getting new blood to put into the system.

C. Robert Valeri: Yes.

Celso Bianco: Do you know any system or any place that uses frozen blood as part of managing their inventory, except for big emergencies or within the military?

C. Robert Valeri: I can't answer that. I don't know.

Alvin Drake: Wasn't there a period when the Cook County Blood Bank had a student of Charles Huggins, who tried to run a 100 percent frozen blood operation?

C. Robert Valeri: Yes. That was Gerald Moss. When he returned from Vietnam, he went to Cook County and for a period of one to two years, ran the Cook County Blood Bank using frozen deglycerolized red cells.

Alvin Drake: Why would they do that?

C. Robert Valeri: If you read the early papers on the work by the Navy, the purpose was not to use frozen red blood cells exclusively, but to use them as a supplement to the liquid blood banking system.

Alvin Drake: He had some kind of disinfection procedure?

C. Robert Valeri: The original concept by James Tullis was that when glycerol was added and removed from red blood cells during the freezing procedure, the virus associated with hepatitis was eliminated. The primary goal of frozen deglycerolized red blood cells in those days was to provide hepatitis-free red blood cells.

Joseph Fratantoni: The use of deglycerolized red blood cells to prevent the transmission of hepatitis was not confirmed by several published reports.

C. Robert Valeri: Harvey Alter, Harold Meryman, and others reported that infected chimpanzees whose red cells were frozen, thawed and washed were shown to transmit hepatitis. In addition, R.K. Haugen from Miami, Florida, has published a paper in the *New England Journal of Medicine* which reported that the use of frozen deglycerolized red cells was associated with the transmission of hepatitis. So, as Dr. Fratantoni points out, published papers show that frozen, deglycerolized red blood cells do transmit hepatitis.

Logistical Concerns in Prepositioning Frozen Blood

Michael J. Ward

The Armed Services Blood Program Office, where I have been director for a little over three years, and the Department of Defense are the primary users of frozen blood, so what I want to do today is give you just a little bit of an overview of the Armed Services Blood Program before turning to the topic of frozen blood itself, because our perspective is unique. The reason we use frozen blood differs from that of anyone else in this audience. I think that needs to be said up front.

I am going to focus on four areas very quickly for you: our mission, our distribution system, the frozen blood program, and finally, how we do it. Our office coordinates the blood programs of all three military departments, each of which has a separate FDA license. We make certain that quality blood products, blood substitutes, and blood services are provided.

Over the years we have put a lot of dollars into research and development to make sure that we had what we needed to assist health care providers on the battlefield. Many of you have reaped the benefit of those dollars invested. We have done that for one reason, and that is to make sure our beneficiaries have what they need in peace, peacekeeping, what is now called Operations Other Than War, such as in Haiti and Somalia, and, of course, full-blown war.

We have Army, Air Force, and Navy blood donor centers, but we also have contingency contracts with the American Red Cross and the American Association of Blood Banks (AABB). Those contracts were activated once during Operation Desert Shield in December, before the attack on the Iraqi forces in Kuwait. We have a number of memoranda of understanding with different organizations throughout the United States to supply some of the blood products for our peacetime needs.

All of those blood products, whether collected in-house or provided through memoranda of understanding, are tested in complete accordance with FDA and AABB requirements, and in terms of contingency support, they are shipped to what we call an Armed Services Whole Blood Processing Laboratory

(ASWBPL). Those shipments may then go overseas. We have a unique distribution issue compared to the distribution problems of all of you in here, because we ship internationally as well as nationally.

Blood products go through either a transshipment or a transportable transshipment center. We need to be able to go anywhere in the world. Once the blood products are received at an overseas blood transshipment center, they are stored, transferred to another blood transshipment center, shipped to a blood product depot for long-term storage, or shipped nearer to the front to be held at a blood supply unit. A blood product depot is a frozen blood depot. A blood supply unit is just a regional distribution area, which then sends the blood products down to the using facility. These are medical treatment facilities in all their different sizes and shapes, including ships at sea. The Marines have a unique system that they use as well.

That basically gives you an overview. The ASWBPL is a key linchpin in our system through which all blood is shipped. During Operation Desert Storm many of your centers shipped blood in support of that operation. That blood went first to the ASWBPL at McGuire Air Force Base, New Jersey, a tri-service (Army, Navy, and Air Force) facility operated by the Air Force. It receives and does a final ABO and Rh check on all units of blood before they go overseas. The blood they receive is fully processed, but the reason that final check is done is because that blood may go down to the combat level. If it is labeled as Group O negative, we may infuse it as Group O negative at the combat level without rechecking it. Above the combat level, our hospitals will do full crossmatching before transfusing.

We have built a new Armed Services Whole Blood Processing Center at Travis Air Force Base, California, to take care of our needs in the Pacific. We have renamed the two labs ASWBPL-East, at McGuire, and ASWBPL-West, at Travis. Back in the mid-1980s, with the Russian bear looking at us, we were building the capability to store 50,000 units of frozen red cells at ASWBPL-East. With downsizing, the fall of the Berlin Wall, and the many other political things that have since happened, that number has been tremendously reduced and we have nowhere near that inventory.

The actual frozen red cell units are processed using the Valeri technique—the modified Meryman technique. We use a cardboard box for storage and shipping. We find it is the most resilient in terms of shipping with minimum breakage. We have shipped it all over the world, even to Saudi Arabia during Desert Storm, and had very little problem with breakage.

We can store about 700 units of frozen blood in one of our freezers. The freezer has a double compressor system, so in case one compressor system breaks down the freezer will still operate. When you have 700 units of blood at over a $100 per unit, you don't want to lose it. We do keep out aliquots of each unit in cryovials, so every time a test is added, we pull out those cryovials and retest. If we don't have a sample remaining for testing, the unit gets chucked. In the frozen state that blood may be shipped directly to a blood product depot, which may be located overseas. The important point is that we have frozen blood at both of those Armed Services Whole Blood Processing Laboratories in the United States, one on the East Coast and one on the West Coast.

Should there be a national disaster in which civilian blood centers would require assistance, that blood could be provided from those depots. However, the main thrust is to get it overseas, and that is where the 20 years or the 10 years of storage life becomes very important. When you invest the expense of flying frozen blood from one part of the world to the opposite side, you don't want to do that any more often than you need to. Any extension on the shelf life is critically important to us.

There are frozen depots located in different parts of the world. For example, we have one in Okinawa, Japan. It is a blood donor center as well as a frozen depot, and it is run by the Navy. The depot manager there is also the manager of the entire Pacific blood program for the Department of Defense (DoD). That is a big area of distribution, and he manages all the products for the military within that system. At the Okinawa facility, we can store 10,000 units. Korea is still the hottest game in town. We continue to have a frozen blood program because we are not sure what the North Koreans are going to do, and frozen blood is essential to make sure that we are ready should they decide this is the time to come south.

The current system has two primary drawbacks. One is that it is manpower intensive. With training, one individual can operate four deglycerolizing machines simultaneously, but he or she can only take off one unit per hour from each of those four machines. It takes an awful lot of these instruments and a lot of manpower to rapidly deglycerolize a lot of blood. The second drawback is that when that unit comes off the machine, it is only good for 24 hours. Now, we know based on DoD studies that we could stretch it to 72 hours without any trouble, and if it is a matter of that person losing his life or getting a unit of blood, it can be retained for 72 hours in a combat situation, and we will give the unit. We are going to go with it if we have to, but that is only the last-ditch effort.

I might add at this point that the frozen supply and all the instrumentation that goes into that is only to get us through until the liquid pipeline opens up. We intend to meet all of our wartime requirements with liquid supplies if at all possible. That is what we did in the Persian Gulf. We met the needs there over several months with about 88,000 units of blood going overseas during Operations Desert Shield and Desert Storm, and the vast majority of that was liquid blood. So, when we have time, that is the system we will use. However, frozen blood is our stopgap. In the event of casualties in Korea, for instance, for the first week frozen blood may be all we have. If we didn't have frozen blood, we could not be sure that our people would get the blood that they need.

The numbers have drastically changed in the past few years. With the Soviet Union as our main threat before the fall of the Berlin Wall, we needed to preposition 225,000 units of blood worldwide. That has dropped down to 67,000 units, the bulk of which is in the Pacific, just in case we need it in the Korean scenario. This is the breakdown for the 67,000 units that have been identified to us: Pacific Command says they need 48,000 of these frozen units. Europe has dropped its requirements down to 6,000. Central Command, which takes in the Persian Gulf area, has 2,000 in position at a classified location in the Middle East ready to use at any time. We have a small contingency supply in Southern Command, which covers Latin and South America, and there presently is none in Atlantic Command, although there may be some put up in Iceland.

That is a total of 56,000 units required. The remaining 11,000 units are at our Armed Services Whole Blood Processing Labs: 8,000 units at McGuire and nearly 3,000 units at Travis. These would be the depots into which the civilian community could tap in the event of a disaster, though the blood, in the frozen state and requiring deglycerolization after thawing, would not be immediately available. Another way to look at it is that of the 67,000 units required, we have shipped over 54,000; 13,000 units are still required. The majority of that has been collected and frozen already and is in continental United States depots awaiting transport overseas. You can imagine the logistics of shipping large amounts of frozen blood, not the least of which is if you ship it on dry ice, the airlines will only take a limited amount because of sublimation and displacement of oxygen. We are thus constrained in the amount of blood that we can ship on military or commercial aircraft at any one time.

Some of those 67,000 units are already starting to creep up on that 10-year shelf life. Thus, it is important that we get the approval from the FDA to go another 10 years for this residual requirement. You have already heard a little bit about where we were on that. We were disappointed that we weren't approved for that extension by the FDA. We understand the concern with contamination, but we are still stuck with a product only good for 24 hours postthaw. As a result, we are working very hard on a thawed blood processing system that will give us a sealed system with an extended postthaw shelf life, beyond five days if possible. In addition, we are making a major effort to look to the future on blood products research and development. A major symposium was held in March 1995 at Andrews Air Force Base in Maryland to try to determine what direction the Department of Defense wants to take on blood substitutes in the future.

Let me conclude by briefly summarizing the advantages and disadvantages of frozen blood. The advantage, of course, is it reduces the peak transportation burden. When we go to war, everybody and his brother is trying to get there, and they are trying to take all their equipment with them. That is not the time to be taking up pallet spaces on aircraft with blood products if we can ship it ahead. It is readily available. It is a quality product. It is just like taking a six-day-old red cell, once we have it deglycerolized. It is an excellent product. It just takes awhile to get it to that point. Once the initial investment is made, you are in good shape.

There are several disadvantages to frozen blood, however. It is very expensive to process and it requires these -80°C freezers, which are heavy, bulky, and expensive, although they seem to operate quite well. The deglycerolization is slow and manpower intensive, and postthaw shelf life is currently only 24 hours.

Should you require some of that frozen blood from the military or from the federal government because of a civilian disaster, you would go through the Federal Emergency Management Agency (FEMA). FEMA in turn would contact the Department of Defense. There is an official within the Department of Army, in the Directorate of Military Support, whose responsibility it is to coordinate all of the DoD response to federal disasters. We have had quite a few of those over the last few years, and I am pretty proud of the responses that the military has made in each of those situations. Fortunately, we did not have to provide blood products to Oklahoma City in the wake of the recent bombing. I hope that we'll always have that tremendous outpouring of donor support in the face of such disasters and that, like most insurance, our frozen blood depots won't ever be necessary.

QUESTIONS/COMMENTS

Alvin Drake: In an emergency situation, are you going to be transfusing without crossmatching much of the time?

Michael Ward: Not necessarily. It depends on where the location is. We have hospitals at different levels that range in capability from providing full restorative care down to the emergency assistant, with just the physician only. When we get down to that furthest forward level, it will be Group O uncrossmatched. Everywhere from there back will be fully crossmatched.

Alvin Drake: But then wouldn't I be wishing that I could unfreeze and process in units much bigger than one?

Michael Ward: Oh, absolutely.

Alvin Drake: Isn't there machinery to do that?

Michael Ward: Not yet. The problem is there is no market for it. If this group were to say that the answer to the blood problem in America is that it all needs to be frozen, you would suddenly have a lot of companies very interested in producing a machine that will do what you want. There are some companies out there now, but not the major companies, because it is economics. If a private company cannot see the economic feasibility of doing it, the Department of Defense isn't going to foot the entire bill. There has to be some venture capital that goes into it.

However, we are confident that once this new system comes out and we have the 21 days to work with, then when we see signs that there is going to be a military action, we will begin deglycerolizing and then stockpiling the refrigerators with liquid blood.

C. Robert Valeri: With regard to Al Drake's question about the desirability of thawing and processing in quantities larger than a unit at a time, are you going to get both units from the same individual or are you going to pool units across donors prior to freezing? Right now everybody is actually collecting a single unit of red cells from a donor.

Alvin Drake: Well, if you are going to give me six units in a hurry, I can't believe you are going to get them from the same person, so it won't make much difference if it gets pooled before storage or pooled in me.

Michael Ward: We can deglycerolize more than one unit in a disposable package, and we do do that. The problem, of course, is that you then get into problems with cross contamination. America wants its sons and daughters treated just like you treat them in these civilian hospitals, and that is our goal: to provide the same quality care that they could get if they went to a civilian facility.

Eve Lackritz: If I understand correctly, when you are in a war situation, you import all your blood from the United States. The Saudis didn't donate?

Michael Ward: That is correct. There are some reasons for that. To be politically sensitive, not all of the blood that is available in the world is as good as the blood that we can provide. We want to make sure that all the blood we use meets the same standards, the same level of testing. When we ship a unit of blood, we want the standard of medical care to be identical to that provided in the United States. That way we are assured that all the testing that we require has been done and that they are getting a quality product.

Eve Lackritz: You said you keep an aliquot of blood on all your frozen blood. Do you also keep aliquots from all your regular blood?

Michael Ward: We do, as all blood banks do, but because of the shelf life, 35 to 42 days, those are only kept for a short period of time.

Eve Lackritz: You just keep that extra aliquot for retesting?

Michael Ward: That is right. Only in case we need to do additional tests.

Extended Liquid Storage of Red Blood Cells

John Hess

I was asked to talk about the feasibility and utility of extending the shelf life of red blood cells (RBC). In a sense we could have seven-week red blood cells now. Two years ago, the Federal Republic of Germany licensed PAGGS-mannitol as an additive solution for the seven-week storage of red blood cells collected in standard citrate-phosphate-dextrose (CPD). This solution does not meet the letter of the U.S. requirements for licensure because the in vivo recovery of those cells was 74.6 percent and the U.S. rules require 75 percent. However, the Germans licensed this solution in the context of a national constitutional crisis over sending German soldiers to join the United Nations relief expedition in Somalia and their perception of a national need for better blood storage solutions to be able to provide international blood support.

Claes Högman and his colleagues,[7] who developed the standard European six-week storage solution of saline, adenine, glucose and mannitol (SAGM), have produced an improved version called Research Additive Solution 2 (RAS2) that unequivocally stores packed red cells for seven weeks. Red cell survivals were almost 80 percent after seven weeks of storage. In form, function, and format this solution is similar to the additive solutions that are used in the United States today. It delivers packed cells in 100 ml of additive solution. This solution formulation, which is already owned by one of the major blood bag suppliers in the United States, could be licensed and manufactured, tested, and made available in this country within a period of two years.

Even longer storage is possible. Tibor Greenwalt and his associates have published a description of a solution called Experimental Additive Solution 25

---

[7] Högman, CF, L Eriksson, J Gong, AB Högman and JM Payrat (1995). Shall red-cell units stand upright, lie flat or be mixed during storage—in vitro studies of red cells collected in 0.5 CPD and stored in RAS2 (erythrosol(R)). *Transfusion Science, 16(2):* 193–199.

(EAS-25) that allowed 73 percent survival of packed red cells at nine weeks.[8] The problem with this particular solution is that it requires 200 ml of the additive in the packed red cell unit. This means that the hematocrit of the resulting "packed" cells will only be about 40 percent. Further, the resulting RBC units still contained about 1 percent glycerol. They may not be safe in certain massive transfusion situations. Such a situation would require rethinking how we use red cells. The U.S. Army is currently supporting Greenwalt's testing of our new variants of this solution.

About a decade ago, Harry Meryman and his colleagues[9] showed that human red blood cells can be stored in hypotonic solutions for periods as long as 35 weeks and yield recoverable cells. This technology has been licensed and Bayer has produced a set of derivative solutions. AS-24 is one. The solution performed well in studies done in vitro. We have a cooperative research and development agreement with Bayer to test it in human beings in our lab.

I have reviewed the products pending in the immediate future. Certainly, the potential that Meryman has shown for longer-term storage suggests that there would be a major benefit to understanding the red cell storage lesion. In all likelihood we can extend blood storage even longer.

Extending storage is a useful thing to do. If we had longer liquid red cell shelf life, we could reduce outdating. If we are outdating somewhere between a half million and a million units annually and we can extend the shelf life by one to two weeks, then realistically we can recover somewhere on the order of a hundred to several hundred thousand units of blood a year. That means that over the course of our lifetimes, we can expect to save 10 million units of blood, a billion dollars. Thus, improved storage would pay for itself. Extending the shelf life to seven or eight weeks would mean that blood collected before students went home for Thanksgiving would still be available in January. This has the potential to reduce some seasonal shortages.

My own background as a Battalion Surgeon in Korea, a Support Command Surgeon in Thailand, Director of Health in American Samoa, and a Public Health Service officer on an Indian reservation in the Dakotas, has taught me that the problems of blood storage are worst in isolated places. Those problems are with maintaining inventory. The small size of the population you are serving makes swings in inventory longer and the outdating problems worse. Increased storage life means the ability to rotate stocks between a

---

[8] Dumaswala, UJ, NL Bentley and TJ Greenwalt (1994). Studies in red blood cell preservation. 8. Liquid storage of red cells in a glycerol-containing additive solution. *Vox Sanguinis, 67(2):* 139–143.

[9] Meryman, HT, ML Hornblower and RL Syring (1986). Prolonged storage of red cells at 4 degrees C. *Transfusion, 26(6):* 500–505.

central supplier and the outlying area. It means it is possible to keep blood on hand in outlying areas but still bring it back and utilize most of it.

There is another benefit of improved red cell storage. Blood deteriorates at a fixed rate in a storage solution. If you can improve that storage solution, then the quality of the cells at any given time will be better. This benefits everybody who gets transfused. It is not known if better cells will ever be a material contribution to the economics of transfusion, but they certainly improve care.

Finally, one of the limits of autologous use in this country is the limited ability to draw enough units to meet some kinds of surgical demand. Extending the liquid storage of red cells will improve the availability of autologous blood to people who want it and, therefore, free up allogeneic blood for other uses.

I would like to end this with a plea to support improved storage. Groups such as this Forum can help in several ways. One is to declare that extending storage is useful. Then, researchers and companies who seek resources to improve storage will find them more easily.

Second, groups such as this Forum can certainly encourage good science. Understanding the red cell storage lesion can potentially lead to major benefits.

Third, we should encourage appropriate development. There are many schemes for increasing the storage period of red blood cells. Only some of them are compatible with most uses. What we don't need is more different kinds of blood products. If we are going to improve the storage length of blood, it needs to be compatible with all of the present uses.

Finally, please encourage regulatory approval. Encouraging our colleagues who regulate to hold conferences that address these issues and to publish points to consider is useful.

QUESTIONS/COMMENTS

Celso Bianco: How do you plan to deal with the problems of bacterial contamination?

John Hess: I don't know of any evidence that bacterial contamination at 42 days or 56 days is worse than at 38 days. Steve Wagner and colleagues[10] have recently published a nice review of this whole area, but the problem is uncommon with red blood cells, and when it occurs it is most commonly seen at about 27 days. If a unit is going to be contaminated by psychrophiles

---

[10] Wagner, SJ, LI Friedman and RY Dodd (1994). Transfusion-associated bacterial sepsis. *Clinical Microbiology Reviews, 7:* 290–302.

(bacteria capable of growing at 0–4°C) at 42 days or beyond, it is already grossly contaminated at 27 days.

We are looking at the idea of testing for bacterial contamination and have supported work on devices such as "through the bag" sensors. As you know, we all currently rely on visual inspection at the time of use as our screen for bacteria. People have ideas of measuring the oxygen content by scanning spectrophotometry, and have devised sensors for carbon dioxide, for pH, and for ammonia that can be glued on the outside of the bag. As the ammonia diffuses through it develops a diazo dye that turns black. A calibrated series of these dots that turned black at weekly intervals might be useful for picking up bacterial contamination. We are looking at these, although we don't have any answers yet.

Overview of Blood Substitutes

Joseph Fratantoni

Blood substitute is the name that most people tend to use for materials that are designed to replace red cells. Another name is artificial blood. The military has referred to the material that they would like to develop as a resuscitation fluid, reflecting their primary need to deal with hemorrhagic shock. Probably red cell substitute is the most appropriate name, but from habit we will probably be calling them blood substitutes more often.

The generic name is actually oxygen carriers, and while we talk about using red cell substitutes for hemorrhagic shock or perhaps perioperative hemodilution, there have been other uses. I will talk a bit about one material that was approved for use in perfusing the myocardium during angioplasty, but there are some other possible uses that have been proposed should an oxygen carrier that is safe and effective be developed.

A major problem that we face in evaluating these materials is determining efficacy. It is clear with a number of preparations that they can carry oxygen. We know that there is limited intravascular half-life. Determining criteria for clinical benefit is really a problem. It is difficult to determine when someone needs red cells or when someone benefits from red cells, and it is even more difficult to determine when that person needs a red cell substitute or would benefit from a red cell substitute.

With many of the preparations, the major problems to date have been related to safety. However, you really can't separate the safety problems from the efficacy problem because you will be talking about giving patients a substitute for a product which already is, as we all know, rather safe and effective.

It might be worth thinking for a minute about what the red cell does before trying to replace it. It permits a high hemoglobin concentration by shielding hemoglobin from the high viscosity and oncotic pressure of the vasculature. It allows the hemoglobin to circulate longer, instead of being cleared rapidly by the kidneys.

We have also learned in the last several years that the red cell protects the body from hemoglobin as well as vice versa. Hemoglobin is both a pharmacologically active material and a very tender molecule. Red cells maintain the hemoglobin in a functional state. It is worth recalling that all land-dwelling vertebrates have their oxygen carriers wrapped in a membrane. Trying to strip that membrane away and infuse hemoglobin is a tricky job.

The use of hemoglobin itself is one basic approach, using either human or non-human hemoglobin or the human hemoglobin gene expressed in a recombinant system. It is then modified by cross-linking the subunits of hemoglobin, polymerizing the material so that it circulates for a longer time and it is more stable, conjugating it to macromolecules or encapsulating it within a liposome. The product would then be a modified or encapsulated human or nonhuman hemoglobin.

The use of fluorocarbons is a second approach. They are manufactured and then modified by emulsifying them. The final product is a perfluorocarbon emulsion.

Baxter is working with a cross-linked preparation that is derived from human red blood cells. The Army is working with a very similar product, Biopure, in a joint venture with Upjohn, using bovine hemoglobin from shed bovine blood that is chemically modified.

Northfield Laboratories has human material that is chemically modified and polymerized. Somatogen, in a joint venture with Eli Lilly, has human recombinant material that is expressed in *Escherichia coli* and is additionally modified and cross-linked at the oxygen binding site. Enzon has a polyethylene glycol-conjugated material.

One mechanism for hemoglobin problems that have been seen, which have included hypertension and a number of vasospastic and perhaps musculoskeletal problems, is that hemoglobin not in the red cell is free to diffuse outside the intravascular space and into the vessel wall, where the endothelial cell is releasing an endothelium-derived relaxing factor, now known to be nitric oxide. Nitric oxide will interact with G proteins to form more guanosine monophosphate (GMP), which in turn leads to vascular relaxation. When hemoglobin gets within this vascular wall (and it can do that when it is not encapsulated in a red cell), it will bind nitric oxide even more avidly than it binds oxygen. Without nitric oxide to stimulate GMP formation you don't get vasorelaxation; instead, you get vasoconstriction, which could explain the hypertension and some of the muscular effects that are being seen.

Another possible problem is whether or not hemoglobin is going to deliver oxygen as advertised. Winslow and his co-workers, in studies with hamsters progressively hemodiluted with a hemoglobin solution, have measured the amount of oxygen that is actually delivered to tissue. Hamsters were infused with either hemoglobin or with Dextran. As you hemodilute with Dextran, you get a little more oxygen carried as the dilution decreases viscosity, and then there is a sharp drop in oxygen as dilution increases.

The surprise in this experiment was that with hemoglobin dilution you also get an increase in oxygen delivery for awhile and then a drop. The exact reason for this is still not clear. These results are submitted for publication and I think still being discussed rather intensively. One mechanism that is proposed is that oxygen from hemoglobin is being consumed by the vessel wall. Whatever the mechanism, if this sort of phenomenon turns out to be something that can be repeated by other laboratories, it certainly casts some question about how much good we will ultimately do by infusing hemoglobin solutions.

Perfluorocarbons have also been investigated. Much interest was stimulated by early pictures of a mouse that was submerged in a beaker of perfluorocarbon liquid that had been saturated with oxygen but was still awake and active. The mouse extracts the dissolved oxygen from the liquid the way a fish extracts dissolved oxygen from water.

Perfluorocarbons do not bind oxygen selectively as hemoglobin or red cells do; fluorocarbons simply dissolve the oxygen. Perflubron is a second generation perfluorocarbon which carries more oxygen per amount of oxygen in the air than the first-generation compounds. It can dissolve more oxygen and can itself be more highly concentrated in an emulsion. The fluorocarbons are unusable with water, so, in order to infuse them, you have to put them into an emulsion form.

Perfluorocarbons were developed in the United States in the mid-1960s and tested first clinically by the Japanese in the late 1970s. Then some clinical studies in the United States showed that there really was not any clinical benefit to severely anemic individuals, and a 1983 request to use this material as a blood substitute was not approved. However, in 1989 a perfluorocarbon was approved for selective use for perfusing angioplasty catheters. The market really did not support that material, and production was halted in about 1993. People have thought that the perfluorocarbons may be useful for perfusing ischemic tissues distal to an obstruction, since an emulsified particle of perfluorocarbon is much smaller than a red cell and so might be able to get to places that red cells could not.

One of the problems with perfluorocarbons as a class is that it appears there does seem to be a somewhat dose-related thrombocytopenia that occurs. A research study by Bob Kaufman at Hemagen showed that a few days after the animal received the material, the platelet count went down from about 230 to about 120. This is a problem that is being looked at, although the clinical importance of this is something that is being debated.

Demonstrating efficacy is certainly a challenge that people are looking at right now. A number of possible approaches are being considered. Obviously, you can show that these materials carry oxygen, or you can show that if you infuse hemoglobin, you increase the hemoglobin level, but that does not appear to be a very important end point. One can try to show that they are equivalent to red cells, but we have heard earlier that it is hard enough to show that red cells work.

People are therefore looking for some sort of useful or practical benefit to an organ or to an organism. One possibility is showing that you can decrease allogeneic blood transfusions. Even though we know that the risk of allogeneic transfusion is very low, that might be something that could be considered of benefit and could support approval of such products.

In order to make these demonstrations of efficacy a bit easier, people are looking at different levels of use, localized perfusion, hypovolemic shock, and perioperative hemodilution, trying to go one at a time rather than get approval for all indications at once.

In conclusion, a red cell substitute appears feasible. There has been an enormous amount of research done in the past several years, and major advances have been made. However, progress has been slow. There have been toxicities, and there is still a lack of fundamental information. There was not the same enormous investment in all areas of basic research in the 1970s as there was in the molecular biology that spawned the biotech industry. When the AIDS crisis gave new stimulus to the development of blood substitutes in the 1980s, there was a large infusion of industrial activity.

The military has been interested in red cell substitutes since the late 1970s or early 1980s and has been the mainstay of support for research. Nevertheless, it remains difficult to demonstrate efficacy. The nature of a successful product is going to depend upon the results of our future research, and it may well be that a successful product will be part of an overall approach to the avoidance of allogeneic transfusion.

V
CLOSING REMARKS

Henrik H. Bendixen

Chair, Forum on Blood Safety and Blood Availability

I will make just a few comments and then share the podium with Harvey Klein, who had a lot to do with putting this program together. My most important visual experience having to do with blood, undoubtedly, was watching television the day of the explosion in Oklahoma City, seeing the enormously long lines of people who insisted on donating their blood. This took place not only in Oklahoma City but also in other parts of the country. This brings to mind also the comment that the best place to store the blood reserves is in the body, and with modern transport possibilities, it would seem that in this country our reserves are fairly safe and adequate.

What is striking is how closely the need is being met, and with a relatively small reserve capacity at any given time. What came across was the considerable pride that many of you have in having learned to manage, predict, and meet the changes in demand.

The discussion about importers and exporters was very interesting. Again, it is a question of learning how to manage. At this point it still has the component of competition as far as I can see, but which, at least in the eyes of some, should and will lead to collaboration rather than competition.

I asked about cost because it is very tempting to consider the high cost of establishing modern blood processing centers. You can't help but ask how many such processing centers this country needs. The more we learn to manage the import-export business, it seems to me the fewer such processing centers we shall need.

It would be very interesting to know a great deal more about donor motivation. Clearly, one sore point is donor management. To use a bad metaphor, a blood donor is a gift horse receiving the most extensive dental examination imaginable. There is a contradiction built into the gift relationship, and the necessary concern about the safety of a unit of blood, which increases the need to manage that interface in the best possible way.

The military's capability of storing many units is very important for its purposes. We can all join in the fond hope that the ultimate use of this reserve will be as a backup for civilian catastrophes rather than military operations.

About blood substitutes, only one comment: blood and blood products have become, if not perfectly safe, yet so relatively safe that it is not going to be easy for blood substitutes to compete because these substitutes will be held to the same standards as the current product.

Harvey Klein
Workshop Moderator

I would like to close our workshop by reiterating a few of the important points we heard today. For example, we heard about the current status of the blood supply. Doug Surgenor reported on the most recent data, those available from 1992, which indicated that more than 12 million units were collected by regional blood centers and hospitals in the United States. It was a little distressing to hear that major changes took place in both the collection and transfusion practices from 1989 through 1992, but no one sitting in this room can really tell us what the trends have been from 1992 through 1995. Clearly, that is something we need to work on because we can't address the problems unless we know what the trends are.

We heard about a 7 percent drop in allogeneic collections between 1989 and 1992, but a 9 percent drop in transfusions and a 70 percent increase in autologous blood collections. Only about half of that autologous blood is used, something that, again, should be somewhat distressing for most of us.

That is the story for red cells. We know far less about the other blood components, although we do know that during that same period of time single-donor platelet collections increased 75 percent. We also know that there are about 1.9 million units of blood that are unaccounted for in the United States. It would be nice to account for those units and to know whether those are units that actually could be recovered for transfusion somehow or whether those are units that are inevitably lost by breakage, by outdating that can't be addressed, and perhaps by mismanagement or units that are of the wrong blood group.

Dr. McCullough then carried on this theme, telling us that inadequate supply leads to danger to patients, and perhaps increased costs due to longer hospitalizations and postponed surgeries. However, excess collection of blood also leads to increased costs. Dr. McCullough also showed us data concerning the fluctuations of blood collections and blood use both at the University of Minnesota and nationally. He pointed out that with data collection by month to month, one couldn't really say much about the fluctuations except that perhaps there were some. I thought it very interesting that while the average weekly usage at the University of Minnesota was 264 units, the range was 195 to 395 per week and that one couldn't really predict what collections would be. He also speculated on why there might be problems with collections, and it was impressive to me that there were no data as to what these reasons were.

Dr. Carson addressed the impossible question, which is whether blood is being used appropriately in the United States. He told us about mortality and morbidity during surgery and questioned whether they could be changed by transfusion. He discussed the increased morbidity and mortality in the Jehovah's Witnesses that one sees with falling hemoglobin concentrations and with cardiovascular complications. We don't know whether transfusion would correct mortality, and this cries out for controlled studies. We can only hope that those might be carried out, given the current financial situation of some of our sources of research funding. That, too, appears to be somewhat of a problem.

Dr. Westphal cautioned us not to treat donors as "reagents." And he pointed out some of the differences in the blood systems in Western Europe and those in the United States. Although his data go back to 1989, it was certainly interesting to see that the Swiss have 100 donors per 1,000 population, while in the United States we have 54. Perhaps that is all we need, but perhaps we need to do better than that if we are to have an adequate blood supply. Dr. Westphal also pointed out that in Switzerland small towns and villages have a sense of community. In the United States, we hear that it may be better to move away from a community responsibility and perhaps move to a more central idea of a national blood supply.

Mr. Bonk told us about the very impressive Delaware Plan: 30 years of no appeals and no shortages. It is a replacement-type plan. Others felt that while that might work in Delaware it probably would not work in Los Angeles or New York City.

Professor Cohen reminded us that if something is valuable the best way to acquire it is to pay for it. There is no such thing as a free lunch, only lunches that others pay for.

Professor Drake told us, again, based on a fair amount of data obtained over a long period of time, that the American blood donor is a marvelous individual. They are out there to donate, if only we need them, and perhaps we don't need them in any greater numbers. Perhaps we are getting as much as we need and we are maintaining a very narrow supply over demand because that is the way our system works. However, the donors are out there. Every year, 10 percent of eligible donors give about 1.5 times a year and that is 3 percent of our population, but, in fact, more than 50 percent of eligible donors have given at some time.

I thought one of the more interesting sessions was the panel on distribution, where first we heard about the Red Cross's Hub system and some of its problems, along with some of its successes. We also heard about the efforts to dissociate the concept of blood as a local community resource and make it more of a national resource. This contrasts with what Dr. Westphal found in a very successful system in Switzerland.

Dr. Simon described to us both United Blood Service's system and the national blood exchange program of the AABB, as well as the problems of providing blood to remote areas.

Dr. Gilcher turned the well-known "triad" on its head, telling us that today, perhaps, cost is more important than availability and more important than quality and safety. I think he didn't really believe that, but hoped to make us think a little bit about what is really important in the national blood supply. He also reminded us of the truism that if a blood center meets hospital needs in all three of those areas, the hospitals will not go elsewhere.

Dr. Bracey gave us the hospital's perspective and let us know that exchange of inventory information is not routine. I think that it was probably surprising to many of us to realize that many hospitals have no idea of what the inventory is for their city, their region, or their state.

I found Mr. Fields' presentation a very interesting one. Kroger buys and ships a billion pounds of perishables annually. That is about the weight of the blood that we ship around annually. His products have a shelf life of 3 to 45 days; again, our platelets outdate at 5 days, and our red cells outdate at 42 days. Perishables are collected locally but shipped and distributed nationally, and availability is controlled by a central clearinghouse. So there are a lot of similarities here between seafood and blood. Kroger has a quality assurance program, and they are, of course, regulated by the FDA, as well as by the USDA and state agencies. They are moving from a hub system to a general distribution system and hope to thereby reduce wastage to 5 to 7 percent. Finally, he told us how using a satellite-type system seems to be effective for moving their perishables around. I can see the large red satellite in the sky now, moving blood around the United States.

Dr. Valeri described cryopreservation of red cells for us. These systems have been useful in a variety of areas, but they do not appear to be very useful for managing the civilian blood inventory on a day-to-day basis in the United States. However, they certainly could be used for potential quarantine problems, for rare blood types, and for some rare medical indications in which freezing is important.

Colonel Ward pointed out to us that freezing blood is very important for the military, and I can only second Dr. Bendixen's thought that we hope that that does apply to the civilian world and we won't need to use those 67,000 units frozen and stockpiled around the world for military casualties.

Colonel Hess pointed out to us that we shouldn't forget about extended storage, refrigerated liquid storage, even though the research in that area has almost disappeared in the last 15 years. A few persistent and successful researchers continue to work in this scientific area. It remains important research that could save several hundred thousand units a year. Extended shelf life certainly could be helpful for remote areas of the United States and for making autologous blood more effective for those individuals for whom it is indicated.

Finally, Dr. Fratantoni told us about the future of red cell substitutes, which may not be quite as close to the horizon as I recently read. We are likely to see such an oxygen carrier within the next several years, however, and perhaps it will find its niche in our blood supply.

In closing, I was most impressed by the diversity of the U.S. system, the systems of collection, of distribution, of inventory control. I think some might be surprised that it works at all. The others will say it works very well and, in fact, only needs a little bit of fine-tuning in order to work almost perfectly.

I thank you all for attention and your comments today, and I hope that we have at least raised a number of issues that will send you home thinking about how we can better make availability less of a problem in the United States.

APPENDIXES

APPENDIXES

A

Acronyms

AABB	American Association of Blood Banks
ABC	American Blood Commission
ABRA	American Blood Resources Association
AIDS	acquired immune deficiency syndrome
ALT	alanine aminotransferase
ARC	American Red Cross
ASWBPL	Armed Services Whole Blood Processing Laboratory
CBER	Center for Biologics Evaluation and Research, Food and Drug Administration
CCBC	Council of Community Blood Centers
CDC	Centers for Disease Control and Prevention
CJD	Cruetzfeldt-Jacob disease
CUE	confidential unit exclusion
FDA	Food and Drug Administration
HBV	hepatitis B virus
HBcAB	hepatitis B core antibody
HCV	hepatitis C virus
HIV	human immunodeficiency virus
HTLV	human T-lymphocyte virus
MI	myocardial infarction
NIH	National Institutes of Health
OBI	Oklahoma Blood Institute
RBC	red blood cells
STS	serologic test for syphilis
USDA	U.S. Department of Agriculture

ACRONYMS

B
Workshop Participants

(Speakers and Forum members are listed separately on pages *iii* and *iv*)

Deidra Abbott
College of American Pathologists

Maj. Janine Babcock, U.S. Army
The Blood Research Detachment
Walter Reed Army Institute of
 Research

Steve Bradshaw
Executive Vice President
Lifeblood

Eileen Church
American Association of Blood Banks

Donald Colburn
American Home Care Federation

Richard J. Davey, M.D.
Chief Medical Officer
American Red Cross

Garth Granrud
Marketing Research
American Red Cross

Liz Hudak
American Red Cross

David E. Jenkins, Jr.
American Red Cross
Louisville Regional Blood Center

Kurt Kroemer
U.S. General Accounting Office

Karen Shoos Lipton, J.D.
Chief Executive Officer
American Association of Blood Banks

Peter Logue
Coral Therapeutics

Jane Mackey, MBA
President
American Association of Blood Banks

James L. MacPherson
Executive Director
Council of Community Blood Banks

Jean Otter, MT (ASCP), SBB
American Association of Blood Banks

Rob Purvis
Blood Center of Southeastern
Wisconsin

James Reilly
Executive Director
American Blood Resources Association

Ernest Simon, M.D.
Executive Vice President
Blood Systems, Inc.

Jennifer Thomas
American Society of Clinical
 Pathologists

Robert Travis
President and CEO of the Blood Bank
 of Delaware